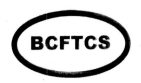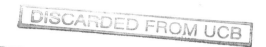

£24.00

BIRMINGHAM COLLEGE OF FOOD, TOURISM & CREATIVE STUDIES
COLLEGE LIBRARY, SUMMER ROW
BIRMINGHAM B3 1JB
Tel: (0121) 243 0055

DATE OF RETURN

Books <u>must</u> be returned by the last date stamped
or further loans may not be permitted

Closed Kinetic Chain Exercise

A Comprehensive Guide to Multiple-Joint Exercise

Todd S. Ellenbecker, MS, PT, SCS, OCS, CSCS
George J. Davies, MEd, PT, SCS, ATC, CSCS

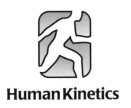

Human Kinetics

Library of Congress Cataloging-in-Publication Data

Ellenbecker, Todd S., 1962-
    Closed kinetic chain exercise : a comprehensive guide to multiple-joint exercise / Todd
S. Ellenbecker, George J. Davies.
        p. cm.
    Includes bibliographical references and index.
    ISBN 0-7360-0170-0
    1. Musculoskeletal system--Diseases--Exercise therapy. 2. Biomechanics. 3. Exercises.
I. Davies, George J.

    RC925.5.E45 2001
    616.7'062--dc21

                                                                                    00-050034

ISBN: 0-7360-0170-0

Acquisitions Editor: Loarn D. Robertson, PhD; **Developmental Editor:** Spencer J. Cotkin, PhD; **Managing Editor:** Sandra Merz Bott; **Assistant Editor:** Sandra Merz Bott; **Copyeditor:** Karen Bojda; **Proofreader:** Jim Burns; **Indexer:** Marie Rizzo; **Permission Manager:** Courtney Astle; **Graphic Designer:** Nancy Rasmus; **Graphic Artist:** Dawn Sills; **Photo Manager:** Clark Brooks; **Cover Designer:** Keith Blomberg; **Photographer (cover):** Russ Adams; Tom Roberts; **Photographer (interior):** Jim Tritch; Todd Ellenbecker; Tom Roberts; **Art Manager:** Craig Newsom; **Illustrator:** Craig Newsom; **Printer:** Edwards Bros.

Printed in the United States of America   10 9 8 7 6 5 4 3 2 1

Human Kinetics
Web site: www.humankinetics.com

United States: Human Kinetics
P.O. Box 5076
Champaign, IL 61825-5076
800-747-4457
e-mail: humank@hkusa.com

Canada: Human Kinetics
475 Devonshire Road Unit 100
Windsor, ON N8Y 2L5
800-465-7301 (in Canada only)
e-mail: hkcan@mnsi.net

Europe: Human Kinetics, P.O. Box IW14
Leeds LS16 6TR, United Kingdom
+44 (0) 113 278 1708
e-mail: humank@hkeurope.com

Australia: Human Kinetics
57A Price Avenue
Lower Mitcham, South Australia 5062
08 8277 1555
e-mail: liahka@senet.com.au

New Zealand: Human Kinetics
P.O. Box 105-231, Auckland Central
09-523-3462
e-mail: hkp@ihug.co.nz

I would like to dedicate this book to the life of Carol J. Davies.
Todd Ellenbecker

Carol J. Davies, 1947-2000
My Hero and Best Friend

Carol J. Davies, my wife, best friend, and soul mate of 32 years, was reborn
into the Kingdom of Heaven on December 20, 2000, in the prime of life.
She passed into Heaven with her loving family at her side. She was her family's
Hero as she courageously fought a rare form of cancer for 3 months. Her sons
Scott and Steven, daughter-in-law Nikki, and granddaughter Lexi, and I were
with her every minute during her 2-week hospice stay at home. Thank you to
the love and strength of our family and friends who helped Carol through the
most difficult thing we have ever had to face together. We provided loving care
to her, and she was an inspiration to us as she demonstrated dignity to the end.
She was a gift from God and forever touched our lives.

Carol was known by everyone as a kind, caring, and compassionate person.
Carol's happiest times were when she was with her family, pet animals,
and friends. She was a fitness enthusiast and a runner for over 20 years.
She participated in many road races over the years and won many trophies.
She practiced a true fitness and wellness lifestyle, including aerobic exercises,
weight training, weight control, appropriate nutrition and diet practices,
and preventive health and medical testing.

She had a wonderful life with her family who she loved very much. Those
who had the opportunity to know her were fortunate and she enriched all
of our lives. Her love, kindness, caring, and compassion will be deeply
missed by family, friends, and all who knew her.

Good-bye to my *Hero* until we meet again.

With love,
George J. Davies
and The Davies Family

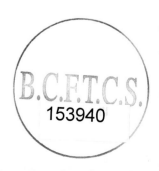

Contents

Acknowledgments

Thanks to Todd for his help with this project, particularly during very difficult circumstances. Todd has been the consummate professional clinician and educator as well as a tremendous contributor to the professional literature. I am proud to be one of his former teachers and to call him one of my protégés. Thanks to Gail for her editorial assistance and continuous support. Thanks to Sandra Merz Bott and the professional staff at Human Kinetics for all their assistance in helping this project come to fruition. Thanks to all patients, students, and professional colleagues who have shared information and themselves to help others.

George J. Davies

Credits

Figure 2.1 Reprinted, by permission, from Palmitier RA, An KN, Scott SG, Chao EY. 1991. Kinetic chain exercise in knee rehabilitation. Sports Med. 11(6):402–413.

Figure 2.2 Reprinted, by permission, from Yack HJ, Collins CE, Whieldon TJ. 1993. Comparisons of closed and open kinetic chain exercise in the anterior cruciate ligament–deficient knee. Am J Sports Med 21(1):49–54.

Table 2.1 Reprinted from Fleming BC, Beynnon BD, Renstrom PA, Johnson RJ, Nichols CE, Peura GD, Uh BS. 1999. The strain behavior of the anterior cruciate ligament during stair climbing: an in-vivo study. Arthroscopy 15(2):185–191.

Table 2.2 Data from Hubley CS, Wells RP. 1983. A work-energy approach to determine individual joint contribution to vertical jump performance. Eur J Appl Physiol. 50:247–254; data from Robertson DG, Fleming D. 1987. Kinetics of standing broad and vertical jumping. Can J Sport Sci 12:19–23.

Figure 2.3 Reprinted, by permission, from Lutz GS, Palmitier RA, An KN, Chao EY. 1993. Comparison of tibiofemoral joint forces during open-kinetic-chain and closed-kinetic-chain exercises. J Bone Joint Surg Am 75(5):732–739.

Table 2.3 Data from Schulthies SS, Ricard MD, Alexander KJ, Myrer W. 1998. An electromyographic investigation of 4 elastic tubing closed kinetic chain exercises after anterior cruciate ligament reconstruction. J Athl Training 33(4):328–335.

Table 2.4 Reprinted, by permission, from Graham VL, Gehlson GM, Edwards JA. 1993. Electromyographic evaluation of closed and open kinetic chain knee rehabilitation exercises. J Athl Training 28(1): 23–30.

Figures 3.1, 3.2, and 3.3 Adapted, by permission, from Groppel JL. 1992. High tech tennis. 2nd ed. Champaign, IL: Human Kinetics, 79.

Table 3.1 Adapted, by permission, from Kibler WB. 1994. Clinical biomechanics of the elbow in tennis: implications for evaluation and diagnosis. Med Sci Sports Exerc 26(10):1203–1206.

Table 6.1 Reprinted, by permission, from Moseley JB, Jobe FW, Pink M, Perry J, Tibone J. 1992. EMG analysis of the scapular muscles during a shoulder rehabilitation program. Am J Sports Med 20(2):128–134.

Table 6.2 Reprinted, by permission, from Kibler WB, Livingston B, Bruce R. 1995. Current concepts in shoulder rehabilitation. In: Advances in operative orthopaedics. Volume 3. St. Louis: Mosby-Year Book. p. 249–297.

Figure 8.1 Reprinted, by permission, from Fleck SJ, Kraemer, WJ. 1987. Designing resistance training programs. Champaign, IL: Human Kinetics, 61.

Introduction

The primary purpose of this book is to provide the clinician and sport scientist with a reference for the application of closed kinetic chain exercise to patients, athletes, and individuals attempting to improve their musculoskeletal conditioning. While many current practitioners working in the medical, health, and sport science arenas have witnessed the recent trend in using closed kinetic chain exercise, the initial popularity of closed kinetic chain exercise and the kinetic chain principle occurred in the late 1800s. Prior to the invention of the isokinetic dynamometer in the 1960s, most rehabilitation and conditioning used traditional closed kinetic chain exercises such as the squat, lunge, and push-up. The isokinetic dynamometer provided a method for open kinetic chain testing and training, allowing clinicians to evaluate and treat isolated muscles and muscle groups. As a result, the dynamometer shifted the trend to use of open kinetic chain training as the state-of-the-art application.

While the use of closed kinetic chain exercise is by no means new or state of the art, only recently has research been published that outlines the effectiveness and general characteristics of this type of exercise. It is the goal of this book to provide the reader with not only the practical tips and guidelines for optimal application of closed kinetic chain exercises, but also the scientific basis, efficacy, and limitations of this type of exercise.

This book begins with an extensive review of the characteristics and biomechanical and physiological principles of closed kinetic chain exercise, as well as a comparison and contrast with open kinetic chain exercise. This is followed by a review of the kinetic chain concept and how it is applied in everyday activities and in sport-related movement patterns. Following the discussion of the kinetic chain concept, the use of closed kinetic chain exercise in rehabilitation and conditioning is illustrated first in the lower extremity and then in the upper extremity (specifically, the shoulder and elbow). The final two chapters provide the reader with a detailed description and illustration of each closed kinetic chain exercise recommended in this text. The goal of these final chapters is to provide an easy-to-use manual with practical applications, proper technique, and indications for closed kinetic chain exercises for patients, athletes, and general populations.

Previous books and articles that discussed closed kinetic chain exercise usually focused on either theoretical aspects or practical applications. This text provides comprehensive scientific background on closed kinetic chain exercise principles as well as a simple, easy-to-use manual for the field or clinic. The blending of practical application and scientific rationale contained in this book provides a detailed base of knowledge for the practitioner in addition to information that can be used in clinical, athletic, and fitness applications.

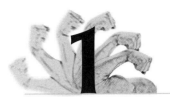

Essential Concepts and Terms

The application of specific exercises for injury rehabilitation and performance enhancement requires a detailed understanding of the underlying characteristics, benefits, and potential consequences of the type of exercise selected. Many of the exercises used in rehabilitation and performance enhancement can be categorized as open or closed kinetic chain exercises. This chapter provides an overview of the kinetic chain principle and the characteristics of open and closed kinetic chain exercise. More detailed descriptions of closed kinetic chain techniques, as well as exercise selection and progression, are the focus of the remaining chapters of this book.

Kinetic Chain Principle

The concept of the kinetic chain, or kinetic link, originates from the area of mechanical engineering. Reuleaux proposed the engineering link concept in 1875 in Heidelburg, Germany, in what has been described as *theoretische kinematik,* or kinematic theory (Gowitzke and Millner 1988; Steindler 1973). In Reuleaux's theory, rigid, overlapping segments were connected via pin joints. These interposing joints created a system whereby movement at one joint produced or affected movement at another joint in the kinetic link.

The conceptual framework proposed in engineering for describing rigid structural elements was adapted by Steindler (1955) and extrapolated to include the analysis of human movement, including exercise and sport-specific activity patterns. Steindler (1955) proposed that the extremities be thought of as rigid, overlapping segments in series; he defined the kinetic chain as a "combination of several successively arranged joints constituting a complex motor unit." These series, or chains, can occur as either of two primary types: open or closed.

Kinetic chain principle describes the body as a series of sequentially activated segments.

Open Kinetic Chain

Open kinetic chain is an exercise or movement pattern where the distal aspect of the extremity is not fixed to an object and terminates free in space.

In an open kinetic chain system, the distal segment of the system or extremity is free to move in space. Using the extremity model, an example of an open kinetic chain would be waving the hand or movement of the foot during the swing phase of gait. Steindler (1955) defined an open kinetic chain as a combination of successively arranged joints in which the terminal segment can move freely. The seated knee-extension exercise is one of the most commonly cited examples of this original open kinetic chain definition (Rivera 1994).

Typically, open kinetic chain exercises are characterized by a rotary stress pattern at the joint. Using the classic example of a seated knee-extension exercise, the rotary stress pattern at the knee involves primarily the rotation of the proximal tibia along the distal femur. While other accessory motions such as tibial rotation and rolling or translation occur (Kapandji 1987), the primary stress imparted to the joint is rotary. Additionally, open kinetic chain movements or exercise patterns occur via one primary axis. For example, the primary-joint instantaneous axis of rotation during the knee-extension exercise is through an evolute of the femoral epicondyle of the tibiofemoral (knee) joint with motion occurring primarily in the sagittal plane.

Evolute is a curve that is the locus of another curve.

Another common characteristic of an open kinetic chain exercise involves the number of simultaneously moving segments. One segment of the joint (i.e., femur in the knee extension) remains stationary during the knee-extension exercise, while the other segment that forms the joint (i.e., tibia) is mobile. This characteristic adds an inherent control to the open kinetic chain exercise movement due to the stability afforded to the stationary segment of the exercising or mobile joint. Open kinetic chain exercises and movement patterns also allow more isolated muscle activation (Palmitier et al. 1991) because such a limited amount of muscular co-contraction is inherent in these exercise movements (Draganich et al. 1989; Palmitier et al. 1991).

While many of the traditionally accepted exercises used in performance enhancement and rehabilitation use open kinetic chain movement patterns or environments, the recent trend has been to include a greater number of closed kinetic chain exercises due to their inherent functional simulation. The primary emphasis of this text is to describe the indications and scientific rationale behind closed kinetic chain exercise. However, the authors recognize the many benefits and indications of open kinetic chain exercise and do not wish to malign in any way this important exercise technique.

Closed Kinetic Chain

Closed kinetic chain is an exercise or movement pattern where the distal aspect of the extremity is fixed to an object that is either stationary or moving.

The definition of a closed kinetic chain exercise or activity that was proposed by Steindler (1955) is a condition or environment in which the distal segment meets "considerable" external resistance that restrains free motion. A system is considered closed when neither the proximal nor the distal segment can move and movement at one segment produces movement or affects motion at all other joints in that kinetic chain in a predictable manner. In Steindler's initial definition, the term "considerable" was not well quantified; this has led to some confusion and controversy over the exact definition of a closed kinetic chain exercise. It is interesting to note that the original engineering definition involved fixture of both the proximal and distal ends of the kinetic link system. In this regard, true closed kinetic chain movement patterns do not technically exist in the human body, except in isometric exercises where no movement of the proximal or distal segments occurs (Dillman et al. 1994; Palmitier et al. 1991; Rivera 1994).

In applying the closed kinetic chain definitions to clinical situations, an exercise in which resistance is placed through the distal aspect of the extremity and remains fixed to the extremity is considered a closed kinetic chain exercise. A primary example of a closed kinetic chain exercise of the lower extremity is a standing squat. In this exercise, the feet remain fixed to the ground during the exercise, and considerable resistance is manifested by the surface as a consequence of the individual's body weight (or added weights in the form of medicine balls or dumbbells). The characteristics of closed kinetic chain environments or movement patterns are listed in table 1.1.

The squat produces a linear stress pattern at the tibiofemoral joint. This pattern is due to the axial joint loading that occurs with weight bearing and closing (fixture) of the distal segment. Movement occurs during the squat at multiple joints using multiple-joint axes at the hip, knee, ankle (talocrural), and subtalar joints. Closed kinetic chain exercise patterns occur with simultaneous movement of both segments that form the utilized joints. This simultaneous and segmental movement causes the increase in muscular co-contraction needed to stabilize and control the movements across the joints in that kinetic link system.

Some exercises, such as the squat or push-up, fall cleanly into Steindler's original definition of closed kinetic chain exercise and involve fixation of the distal segment of the extremity to a load that would qualify as "considerable." However, many common exercises often referred to as closed kinetic chain do not clearly fall into this category. One exercise whose classification as open or closed kinetic chain exercise is uncertain involves stair-climbing machines, where the distal aspect of the lower extremity remains fixed to an object (the pedal) that is constantly moving during exercise. Similarly, riding a bicycle involves a closed system, but many clinicians and researchers argue that the movement of the pedal and the trivial resistance level occasionally encountered while pedaling do not clearly qualify that exercise as a closed kinetic chain exercise.

For the purpose of this book, in a closed kinetic chain exercise, the distal aspect of the extremity is fixed to either a stationary object (such as the ground during a squat or push-up) or a moving object (as with the use of a stair-climbing or

Table 1.1   Characteristics of Open and Closed Kinetic Chain Exercises

Characteristic	Open kinetic chain	Closed kinetic chain
Stress pattern	Rotary	Linear
Number of joint axes	One primary	Multiple
Nature of joint segments	One stationary, the other mobile	Both segments move simultaneously
Number of moving joints	Isolated joint motion	Multiple-joint movement
Planes of movement	One (single)	Multiple (triplanar)
Muscular involvement	Isolation of muscle or muscle groups, minimal muscular co-contraction	Significant muscular co-contraction
Movement pattern	Often nonfunctional movement patterns	Significant functionally oriented movement patterns

elliptical machine). The characteristics listed in table 1.1 are used to qualify the exercises in this text as closed kinetic chain.

Other Commonly Used Terms

Table 1.2 contains some of the terms used to describe exercise or movement patterns commonly applied in both rehabilitation and performance enhancement.

Single-Joint Versus Multiple-Joint Exercise

The terms *single joint* versus *multiple joint* have been used to describe exercises based on the number of joints being exercised, in contrast to the kinetic chain type classification, which considers whether or not the distal aspect of the extremity is fixed (Dvir 1996). Single-joint exercises correspond closely with traditional open kinetic chain exercise movements such as the biceps curl and seated knee extension. These exercises consist primarily of movement at one joint and generally allow isolated joint testing and training (Feiring and Ellenbecker 1996). Single-joint exercises are also commonly referred to as *joint-isolation exercises* because these types of exercises isolate activity at one particular joint and often isolate particular muscles or groups of muscles (Feiring and Ellenbecker 1996).

Multiple-joint exercises correspond closely with exercises that are commonly classified as closed kinetic chain. Movement occurs at multiple levels with muscular co-contraction during these exercises, and the ability to exercise numerous segments and muscle groups simultaneously is their primary benefit (Fleck and Kraemer 1987).

Boundary Condition and Load

Dillman et al. (1994) proposed an alternative method of classifying exercises based on mechanics. They used the boundary condition and the presence or lack of an external load as the two criteria in the classification scheme. The boundary condition is termed either *fixed* or *movable,* rather than closed or open. An external load may or may not exist with the exercise. Therefore, Dillman et al. (1994) proposed three categories of exercise:

- Fixed with external load (FEL), which most closely corresponds with the classic definition of a closed kinetic chain exercise. Examples include the push-up or squat.
- Movable boundary with no external load (MNL). This condition corresponds closely with a true open kinetic chain exercise. Examples are raising the arm or extending the lower leg with no resistance applied.

Table 1.2 Comparison of Terminology in Open and Closed Kinetic Chain Exercise

Kinetic chain	Joint multiplicity	Boundary condition and load
Open kinetic chain	Single joint	FEL (fixed, no external load)
Closed kinetic chain	Multiple joint	MNL (moving, no load)
	Uncertain classification	MEL (moving, external load)

- Movable boundary with external load (MEL). This condition attempts to classify the gray area in the open/closed chain classification and the single-/multiple-joint classification system. Dillman et al. (1994) provided examples that included a bench-press exercise for the upper extremity and a stair-climbing or leg-press exercise for the lower extremity.

These terms may be beneficial in descriptively labeling exercises that do not clearly fit into the more traditional kinetic chain classification system. Blackard et al. (1999) compared the electromyographic (EMG) activity of upper-extremity musculature for the three exercise classifications of Dillman et al. (1994). Blackard et al. (1999) documented similar EMG activity in the upper-extremity musculature during exercise with different boundary conditions. They concluded that the presence of an external load may be more important than the boundary condition when analyzing muscular activity levels during exercise. Further research using this exercise classification system is needed so that it may assist clinicians with the application of exercise to both patients and athletes.

The terms *open* and *closed* kinetic chain have recently come under scrutiny in the physical medicine and rehabilitation arenas (Buckley 1997; DiFabio 1999). The classification of rehabilitative exercise and operational nomenclature have been recently discussed at meetings and in publications (Buckley 1997; DiFabio 1999). Despite the recent debate, we feel that the terminology of open and closed kinetic chain exercise is commonly used, applied, and understood. Therefore, in this text, we use Steindler's (1955) definition of a closed kinetic chain exercise. Further research is needed to more clearly define the effects of different types of exercise on the human musculoskeletal system and possibly generate a more definitive classification system. Until that time, we feel that the present classification system has merit, and we will not belabor the semantic debate over exercise classification. The presentation of alternative methods of exercise classification and terminology is not meant to confuse the reader, but only to identify and inform the reader that alternative methods and theories are currently present.

Electromyographic (EMG) is a measurement technique used to detect discharges of electrical activity from individual motor units in skeletal muscle and provide information regarding the frequency of firing in motor nerve fibers and muscular activity.

Summary

Several key operational definitions in this chapter create the platform for the physiological and biomechanical discussion and the application of the kinetic chain system in upcoming sections of this book. A complete understanding of the critical characteristics of the kinetic chain and of both open and closed kinetic chain exercise will enable optimal application of the exercises detailed later in this book.

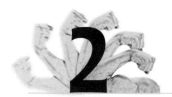

2

Biomechanics and Physiology of Closed Kinetic Chain Exercise

A firm understanding of the biomechanical and physiological principles relevant to closed kinetic chain exercise better allows the clinician to apply this exercise modality. This chapter outlines the primary biomechanical characteristics of closed kinetic chain exercise and discusses the muscular activity patterns and physiological demands on the extremity being exercised.

Biomechanical Principles of Closed Kinetic Chain Exercise

One of the primary biomechanical issues discussed in the literature regarding closed kinetic chain exercise is the stress placed on the ligamentous structures of the knee during movement. Careful comparison between open and closed chain exercise allows the inherent forces and biomechanical features of these exercise classifications to best be understood.

Palmitier et al. (1991) provided force diagrams of the seated knee-extension exercise under different load conditions (figure 2.1). Of particular importance is the size of the shear force (S) in each load condition. The shear force represents stress imparted primarily to the anterior cruciate ligament (ACL). In figure 2.1a, the load is applied to the distal aspect of the extremity in a simulated open kinetic chain knee-extension exercise. Under this condition the shear force is directed posteriorly and is the largest of the four examples. This posteriorly directed shear force produces anterior tibial displacement and stresses the ACL. In the condition illustrated in figure 2.1b, a more proximal point of force application is depicted, significantly decreasing the amount of shear force at the tibiofemoral joint. The condition shown in figure 2.1c demonstrates the effect of an axial load application that simulates the

Shear force is coplanar and opposite in direction but is not colinear; it is a force that causes one surface of a body to slide past an adjacent surface.

type of loading in a closed kinetic chain exercise. Once again, the shear force is minimized through the use of an axial load that compresses the tibiofemoral joint surfaces, which together decrease the shear force. Finally, in figure 2.1d, a hamstring and quadriceps co-contraction is simulated. The posteriorly directed pull of the biarticular hamstrings dramatically decreases the shear force (Palmitier et al. 1991). Coactivation of the hamstrings helps to neutralize the anterior displacement caused by quadriceps contraction and also stabilizes the more proximal hip joint. Closed kinetic chain exercises serve to minimize the tibiofemoral shear forces through both axial loading and hamstring coactivation (Palmitier et al. 1991).

Several studies have been performed that support the force diagrams of Palmitier et al. (1991). These studies attempted to measure the stresses on the ligamentous structures of the knee using both direct and indirect methods. In a classic study, Henning et al. (1985) used a strain gauge in vivo to directly study the forces on the human ACL. Their study used exercise activities such as knee extension with a 20-lb (9 kg) boot in the range of motion between terminal extension and 22° of knee flexion. This open kinetic chain knee-extension exercise produced peak elongation of the ACL at rates of 87% to 121% of the elongation produced with an 80-pound (36 kg) Lachman test. Exercises such as cycling and the one-leg half-squat produced only 7% and 21%, respectively, of the stress imparted with the 80-pound Lachman test. However, Henning et al. (1985) only used two experimental subjects, including one with an ACL-deficient knee.

In vivo—occurring within the living organism.

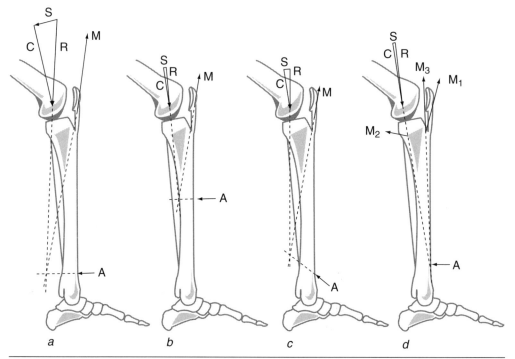

Figure 2.1 The reaction forces at the knee joint are altered by the exercise modality and location of applied force. A = the point/direction of the force application; C = the compressive component of the joint reaction force; M = the simulated muscle forces; R = the joint reaction force; S = the shear component of the joint reaction force. (a) Knee-extension exercise with force applied on distal tibia. (b) Knee-extension exercise with force applied more proximally. (c) Force applied with an axial orientation. (d) Quadriceps and hamstring co-contraction during distal force application.
From Palmitier et al. 1991.

Axial force is a force that is directed along the axis of a joint or bone usually resulting in compression of the joint surfaces together.

Another study that demonstrates the biomechanical principles of closed kinetic chain exercise was done by Yack et al. (1993). They measured anterior tibial displacement in subjects with ACL-deficient knees with an electrogoniometer at three different times: during a Lachman test, during an open chain knee-extension exercise, and during a parallel squat exercise. Results showed significantly greater anterior tibial translation during the open chain knee-extension exercise from 64° to 10° of knee flexion than during the closed chain parallel squat exercise (figure 2.2). These authors attributed the limitation of anterior tibial displacement during the closed kinetic chain parallel squat exercise to the complex interaction of the ligamentous and soft tissue restraints, femoral condylar geometry, active muscle control and co-contraction, and tibiofemoral contact forces. Yack et al. (1993) did not find significant differences in anterior tibial displacement when they studied normal, healthy knees under the same set of experimental conditions.

In a series of in vivo strain gauge studies, Beynnon et al. (1994, 1995, 1997) measured the effects of typical exercises used in both rehabilitation and performance-enhancement programs on ACL strain. Two important findings in these studies were that greater ACL strain occurred during resisted open chain knee-extension exercise than during extension of the knee without an applied load, and that isometric knee extension at 15° and 30° of extension produced significantly greater ACL strain than similar isometric contractions with the knee in 60° and 90°

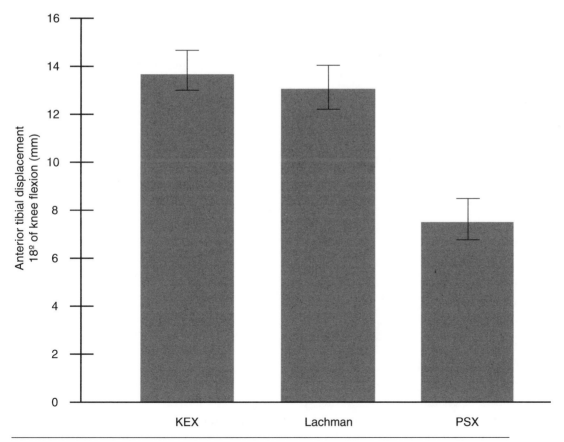

Figure 2.2   Mean anterior tibial displacement and standard error at 18° of knee flexion for the open chain knee-extension exercise (KEX), the Lachman evaluation, and the parallel squat exercise (PSX).

Reprinted from Yack et al. 1993.

of flexion. These authors concluded that exercises that minimize stress to the ACL involve isolated quadriceps activity with the knee flexed 60° or more, simultaneous quadriceps and hamstring activation, or unresisted active knee extension between 35° and 90° of flexion.

In a follow-up study, Beynnon et al. (1997) studied the effects of a closed chain squat exercise on ACL strain, again using an in vivo strain gauge. They found that the strain imparted to the ACL during the performance of a squat with elastic-cord resistance did not significantly differ from the strain to the ACL from a squat without any resistance. Additionally, no significant difference in ACL strain was measured when comparing the closed chain squat exercise with unresisted active knee extension–flexion. Commonly used rehabilitation exercises and their inherent ACL strain are listed in table 2.1, which serves as a valuable resource when evaluating the safety and appropriateness of using these exercises by individuals with compromised ligamentous stability in the lower extremity (Fleming et al. 1999).

In addition to studying shear force and tibial translation, Wilk, Escamilla et al. (1996) measured the tibiofemoral compressive forces during open chain knee-extension exercise and closed chain leg-press and squat exercises. They found

Table 2.1 Rank Comparison of Peak ACL Strain Values During Commonly Prescribed Rehabilitation Activities*

Rehabilitation activity	Peak strain (%)[a]	Number of subjects
Isometric quad contraction at 15° (30 N · m of extension torque)	4.4 (0.6)	8
Squatting with sports cord	4.0 (1.7)	8
Active flexion–extension of the knee with 45-N boot	3.8 (0.5)	9
Lachman test (150 N of anterior shear load, 30° flexion)	3.7 (0.8)	10
Squatting	3.6 (1.3)	8
Active flexion–extension of the knee (no weight boot)	2.8 (0.8)	18
Simultaneous quad and hamstring contraction at 15°	2.8 (0.9)	8
Isometric quad contraction at 30° (30 N · m of extension torque)	2.7 (0.5)	18
Stair climbing	2.7 (2.9)	5
Anterior drawer (150 N of anterior shear load, 90° flexion)	1.8 (0.9)	10
Stationary bicycling	1.7 (1.9)	8
Isometric hamstring contraction at 15° (to –10 N · m of flexion torque)	0.6 (0.9)	8
Simultaneous quad and hamstring contraction at 30°	0.4 (0.5)	8
Passive flexion–extension of the knee	0.1 (0.9)	10
Isometric quad contraction at 60° (30 N · m of extension torque)	0.0	8
Isometric quad contraction at 90° (30 N · m of extension torque)	0.0	18
Simultaneous quad and hamstring contraction at 60°	0.0	8
Simultaneous quad and hamstring contraction at 90°	0.0	8
Isometric hamstring contraction at 30°, 60°, and 90° (to –10 N · m of flexion torque)	0.0	8

[a] Mean (standard deviation)

From Fleming et al. 1999.

significantly higher tibiofemoral compressive force during the closed chain exercise (leg press 5,762 N [newton], squat 6,139 N) than during the open kinetic chain knee-extension exercise (4,598 N). The maximal compressive force occurred at an average of 85° to 95° of knee flexion and at 75° for the open chain knee-extension exercise. Wilk, Escamilla et al. (1996) also reported a posteriorly directed shear force during the closed kinetic chain exercises that peaked at approximately 85° to 105° of knee flexion. This is in agreement with Lutz et al. (1993), who also found posteriorly directed shear forces that create stress in the posterior cruciate ligament with closed kinetic chain exercises such as stair climbing and squatting. The magnitude of the posterior shear forces increased significantly with knee flexion angles greater than 45°.

Biomechanical research provides the clinician with an excellent framework for the use of closed kinetic chain exercise. These studies are invaluable for providing information about the range of motion, the position and direction of resistance application, and its effect on ligamentous structures and tibiofemoral mechanics. Many clinicians deal with individuals with patellofemoral complications (Wilk et. al 1998). Doucette and Child (1996) studied patellar tracking in both open and closed kinetic chain states using computed tomography. They found progressively better patellar tracking in the closed chain, open chain, and relaxed conditions studied as the knee moved from 0° of extension to 40° of knee flexion due to the increased support afforded by the femoral intercondylar groove. Patella tracking became progressively better as the knee moved from 0° of knee extension to 40° of knee flexion for all three conditions studied: closed chain, open chain, and relaxed conditions. In measuring the patellofemoral congruence angle, Doucette and Child (1996) found significantly greater lateral tracking in the open kinetic chain knee extension than in the more medially oriented closed kinetic chain state. The knee-joint range of motion between 0° extension and 40° flexion is where most functional activities take place. In this range of motion, the closed kinetic chain exercise produced better patellofemoral tracking, but open kinetic chain exercise demonstrated greater lateral patellar displacement in these ranges.

Somes et al. (1997) studied the effects of McConnell patellofemoral taping in the open and closed kinetic chain conditions. No significant difference was found in the patellofemoral congruence angle when comparing open and closed kinetic chain taping conditions. Somes et al. (1997) did report larger patellofemoral angles measured with taping in the closed kinetic chain condition, which indicates a more medially tilted patella. This medial tilting was not replicated in the open kinetic chain condition. While further study must be done, it appears that these two preliminary studies demonstrate favorable changes in patellofemoral biomechanics with closed kinetic chain exercises.

One final area of discussion regarding the biomechanics of closed kinetic chain exercise is the functional contribution from adjoining segments in the kinetic chain. This is covered at length in the next chapter, but biomechanical research pertaining to commonly applied closed kinetic chain tests has application in this chapter as well. Table 2.2 lists the relative contributions of the lower-extremity segments during the performance of a vertical jump. Significant contributions from the hip and ankle allow the transfer of force starting from the ground reaction force. This type of research clearly displays the important role of adjoining segments in closed kinetic chain exercises and functional activities where closed kinetic chain environments are used.

One **newton** is defined, in accordance with Newton's second law of motion, as the force acting on a mass of 1 kg that gives an acceleration of 1 meter per second squared (1 newton [N] = 1 kg · m/s²).

Table 2.2 Average Relative Contributions of Lower-Extremity Segments in Vertical Jump Performance

Segment	Hubley and Wells 1983	Robertson and Fleming 1987
Hip	28%	36%
Knee	49%	24%
Ankle	23%	40%

Many clinicians use a horizontal long-jump test, as recommended by the International Knee Documentation Committee (IKDC), to evaluate an individual's lower-extremity function following injury. Robertson and Fleming (1987) also studied the horizontal long jump and found the contributions from the ankle to be 46%; knee, only 4%; and hip, 50%. These numbers indicate that closed kinetic chain testing cannot be used to isolate or measure strength at one joint, but rather to provide the clinician with a whole extremity's functional performance index or parameter.

Moment is the tendency to cause rotation about a point or axis.

Consistent with the findings of Robertson and Fleming (1987), new research published by Ernst et al. (2000) showed significant compensatory activity of the adjoining hip and ankle segments in patients with ACL-reconstructed knees who performed functional movement patterns. This study measured muscular activity and lower-extremity kinetics in patients following ACL reconstructions and a group of age-matched controls while they performed a single-leg vertical jump and a lateral step-up. Relevant findings included significantly reduced knee-extension moments in the ACL-reconstructed limbs when compared with both the uninjured limb and the control-group limbs. However, there was no difference in the summated total leg-extension moment that was created by adding the knee, hip, and ankle moments together. This finding indicates that compensatory activity by the hip and ankle segments occurred to correct for the lack of knee extension during the closed kinetic chain movement patterns studied. These results suggest that the hip and ankle extensors can compensate for the knee-extension deficit that may be present following knee ligament injury. The decrease in knee-extension moment may lead to inadequate attenuation of landing forces during functional movements and may predispose the skeleton and joint structures to injury. This important research provides another example highlighting the potential compensatory activation of the adjoining segments around an injured joint during closed kinetic chain exercise or movement patterns.

In summary, biomechanical analysis of closed kinetic chain exercises has identified several inherent positive benefits for both rehabilitation and performance-enhancement exercise programs, including multiple-joint function, decreased shear force and tibial translation, and more medially oriented patellofemoral positioning.

Physiological Principles of Closed Kinetic Chain Exercise

Similar to the previous section on biomechanical principles of closed kinetic chain exercise, there are inherent physiological principles of this classification of exercise that set it apart from other types or classifications of exercise. One of the most significant physiological characteristics of closed kinetic chain exercise is the multiple-joint and co-contraction muscular activity patterns that produce unique physiological demands and ultimately benefits to the individual performing the activity.

In this section, the physiological demands and characteristics of closed kinetic chain exercise are discussed. One of the main physiological variables discussed is the muscular activity and activation patterns inherent in closed kinetic chain exercises. This discussion of physiological demands and muscular activity patterns will enable the clinician to better understand the inherent demands closed kinetic chain exercises place upon the extremity being exercised.

One of the primary means of analyzing the physiological stresses inherent in closed kinetic chain exercise is through electromyographic (EMG) measurement of muscular activity. EMG, via indwelling and surface electrodes, allows scientists and clinicians to appropriately monitor the muscular activity of muscles and muscle groups during functional activity. Several studies (Lutz et al. 1993; Wilk, Escamilla et al. 1996) using EMG have measured the relative activity of lower-extremity musculature during closed kinetic chain exercise or simulated closed kinetic chain conditions.

Biomechanical research has demonstrated consistently less anterior tibial translation during closed kinetic chain exercise than during exercises or activities performed in an open kinetic chain environment. One of the primary reasons for this decrease in translation of the tibia is the presence of muscular co-contraction during closed kinetic chain exercise. Lutz et al. (1993) used EMG to monitor activity of the quadriceps and hamstrings in subjects performing open chain knee extension, open chain knee flexion, and a closed chain squat exercise. Figure 2.3 displays the results of the EMG analysis, which shows minimal co-contraction (simultaneous activation of the hamstrings and quadriceps) in the open kinetic chain flexion or extension condition. However, during the closed kinetic chain exercise, significant hamstring muscle activity accompanied the predominant quadriceps activity. Of particular interest is the increased amount of hamstring activity measured with the knee joint in 30° of knee flexion, the position where anterior tibial translation and shear forces have been reported to be the highest (Beynnon et al. 1995, 1997; Wilk and Andrews 1993). Lutz et al. (1993) measured sequentially less hamstring coactivation during the closed chain squat exercise as the knee-flexion angle increased from 30° to 90° and concluded that as anteriorly directed tibial translation forces decrease with increased knee flexion, hamstring coactivation also decreases.

Additional EMG research that monitored several lower-extremity muscles has also consistently demonstrated patterns of co-contraction and involvement of the entire lower-extremity musculature during closed kinetic chain activities. The amount of hamstring co-contraction has been consistently documented at less than 20% of maximal voluntary contraction levels, with 12% levels reported by Wilk, Escamilla et al. (1996) during a leg press and 4% to 12% by Isear et al. (1997) during an unloaded squat.

Cook et al. (1992) measured EMG activity of lower-extremity musculature during a lateral step-up and a stair-stepping activity and evaluated the leg-press and squat exercise. While the lateral step-up created significantly greater quadriceps activation levels and the stair-stepping activity caused significantly greater gastrocnemius activity, no significant difference was measured between activities

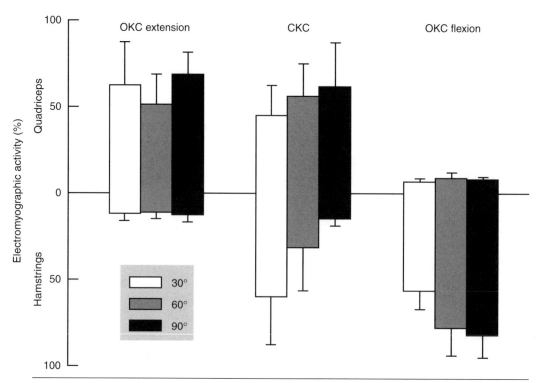

Figure 2.3 The EMG activity of the hamstring and the quadriceps musculature during the open kinetic chain knee-extension exercise (OKC extension), closed kinetic chain squat (CKC), and open kinetic chain knee-flexion exercise (OKC flexion).

Reprinted from Lutz et al. 1993.

in hamstring (biceps femoris, semimembranosus, semitendinosus) activation. The important roles of the biarticular hamstring musculature during closed kinetic chain exercise include stabilizing the hip flexor moment at the hip and secondarily stabilizing the knee joint in resisting anterior tibial translation (Palmitier et al. 1991).

Schulthies et al. (1998) studied the EMG activity in a series of four closed chain exercises using elastic-tubing resistance. These exercises, advocated by many clinicians, consist of multidirectional movements using elastic resistance with unilateral closed chain stance. Schulthies et al. (1998) measured activity of the hamstring and quadriceps musculature during front and back pulls, a crossover, and a reverse crossover maneuver with elastic-tubing resistance attached to the uninjured limb. The limb to be exercised maintains a closed kinetic chain position, while the opposite limb performs resisted movements. Table 2.3 displays the mean muscular activity levels in the quadriceps and hamstring musculature during these elastic-resistance exercises.

Additional research published by Graham et al. (1993) measured the muscular activity of the quadriceps and hamstrings during other closed kinetic chain exercises commonly used by clinicians. Table 2.4 shows the variation in muscular activity and the ratio of activity between the hamstrings and quadriceps during these activities.

Because closed kinetic chain exercise takes place in the lower extremity with the foot firmly attached to a supportive surface and in the upper extremity with the hand attached to a supportive surface or resistant object, it is important to determine optimal positions for placement of the hands and feet during exercise.

Table 2.3 Normalized Mean EMG Values for Four Muscles During Four Elastic-Tubing Closed Kinetic Chain Exercises*

Exercise	VMO	VL	SemiT	BicepF
Front pull	42	36	58	49
Back pull	37	38	13	40
Crossover	31	27	40	27
Reverse crossover	33	35	16	25

* All values are expressed as percentage of maximal voluntary contraction. VMO = vastus medialis obliquus; VL = vastus lateralis; SemiT = semitendinosus; BicepF = biceps femoris.

Data from Schulthies et al. 1998.

Table 2.4 Percentage of Maximal Voluntary Contraction (% MVC) and Hamstrings-to-Quadriceps Ratio (mean ± SD)

	% MVC hamstrings	% MVC quadriceps	Hamstrings/ quadriceps (%)
Fitter	27.2 ± 11.1	38.5 ± 17.4	70.6
Stair-climber	22.6 ± 10.6	36.0 ± 19.7	62.9
Knee extension	18.2 ± 8.6	84.9 ± 29.6	21.5
Quarter squat	15.9 ± 6.4	25.9 ± 6.8	61.5
Slide board	41.3 ± 9.0	55.8 ± 27.3	73.9
Step-up	25.0 ± 8.0	40.9 ± 9.9	61.1

Reprinted from Graham et al. 1993.

To date, no research on upper-extremity closed kinetic chain exercise details hand position relative to extremity rotation and other variables. However, several studies have investigated the effects of lower-extremity axial rotation on EMG activity of the quadriceps and hamstrings during closed kinetic chain exercise. Ninos et al. (1997) studied the Olympic squat maneuver in two positions of lower-extremity axial rotation: a self-selected neutral position and a position termed *turn-out,* in which there is 30° of external lower-extremity axial rotation from the self-selected neutral position. Results of the testing showed no significant difference in vastus medialis obliquus and vastus lateralis activity between the two positions. Additionally, the ratio of vastus medialis obliquus to vastus lateralis activity (or VMO:VL ratio) did not significantly change between positions of axial rotation. No change in hamstring muscular activity was measured as the subjects in this study went from complete extension to 60° of knee flexion in the above kinetic chain. However, the vastus medialis obliquus and vastus lateralis were significantly more active at 40° to 60° of knee flexion than in the arc of motion between 10° and 20° of knee flexion in the closed kinetic chain condition.

Miller et al. (1997a) studied the effects of lower-extremity axial rotation on VMO and VL muscular activity during closed kinetic chain step-ups and modified wall slides. Symptomatic subjects (patients with patellofemoral pain) and asymptomatic subjects were studied using EMG measurement. Results showed no significant effect of leg rotation on VMO:VL for the symptomatic group in either the modified wall slide or step-up/step-down exercise. The asymptomatic group showed lower VMO:VL values with external axial rotation than with neutral and internally rotated positions for the step-up/step-down exercise.

Miller et al. (1997b) published a second study of closed kinetic chain exercise conditions that included a static lunge with 30° and 70° of knee flexion, modified wall slide, and step-up and step-down exercises. Again, no significant difference in VMO activity was measured, but subjects with patellofemoral pain showed greater VL activity and lower VMO:VL ratios during the static lunge exercise with 70° of knee flexion. Further research is needed to better define the role of VMO and VL muscular activity in conjunction with traditionally used lower-extremity exercises. Furthermore, the available studies caution the reader against blindly using only externally rotated foot positions based on unsubstantiated practices or exercise intuition, as no clear effect or improvement in VMO activity is consistently measured with closed kinetic chain exercise using this position. The authors of this book recommend using exercise positions based on scientifically demonstrated principles and individual variation in lower-extremity biomechanics. Because closed kinetic chain exercises involve the entire kinetic chain, the mechanics and potential compensatory deviations during exercise must be closely monitored. While it is beyond the scope of this text to completely review all the biomechanical and physiological variables inherent in human gait, it must be mentioned that evaluation and monitoring of segments proximal and distal to the intended segment of exercise or rehabilitation is imperative when using closed kinetic chain exercise. Using the example of the lower extremity during a squat or lunge, the influence of the subtalar joint during lower-extremity loading and the kinetic chain effects of pronation, including calcaneal eversion and internal tibial rotation, must not be overlooked.

Proprioception is the awareness of joint posture, joint movements, and positional changes.

Afferent receptors are sensory neurons or peripheral receptors present within the muscles, fascia, joint capsule, ligaments, and skin surrounding a joint.

Kinesthesia, often used interchangeably with proprioception, is the ability to discriminate or to perceive joint position, relative weight of body parts, and joint movement, including direction, amplitude, and speed.

One of the other physiological variables that deserves discussion in this chapter is the effect of closed kinetic chain exercise on proprioception. While several mechanisms are responsible for joint proprioception and kinesthesia, the periarticular afferent receptors are an important variable that is affected by both movement and exercise (Rowinski 1985). These periarticular receptors are subject to distortion or stimulation from mechanical forces associated with soft-tissue elongation, relaxation, compression, and fluid tension changes (Rowinski 1985). Afferent mechanoreceptors also work in concert with the muscle spindle system and the vestibular system to provide joint position sense and feedback during movement and exercise (Voight and Cook 1996).

The use of closed kinetic chain exercises, with their inherent compressive and joint approximation characteristics, has been recommended for proprioceptive training following lower- and upper-extremity injuries (Davies and Dickhoff-Hoffman 1993; Voight and Cook 1996). Theoretical increases in afferent receptor activity have been cited as a primary indication for use of closed kinetic chain exercises due to the joint compression and dynamic muscular co-contraction inherent in this type of exercise. The characteristics of closed kinetic chain exercises, including large resistance levels, low accelerations, large compressive forces, enhanced joint congruity, reduced shear force, stimulation of joint proprioceptors, and enhanced dynamic stabilization, make these exercises a popular and effective choice in rehabilitation and performance enhancement (Lephart and Henry 1996).

Rogol et al. (1998) conducted a six-week upper-extremity training study using 39 military cadets (13 performed open kinetic chain exercise, 13 performed closed kinetic chain exercises, and 13 acted as control subjects). They found improved joint reposition sense in the shoulder in both the open and closed chain training groups. These researchers concluded that neither open nor closed kinetic chain exercises were superior; they were both equally effective at enhancing joint reposition sense as compared with the control group that did not exercise.

Summary

The discussion of the biomechanical and physiological characteristics of closed kinetic chain exercise in this chapter highlighted the potential benefits and cautions regarding the use of this exercise modality. Muscular co-contraction, involvement of the entire extremity's kinetic chain, and the neurological benefits of increased proprioceptive and afferent stimulation are some of the advantages discussed in this chapter. Knowledge of the biomechanical and physiological characteristics of closed kinetic chain exercise can lead to improved application of this form of exercise and reinforce the practical presentation of closed chain movement patterns later in this book.

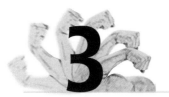

3

The Kinetic Link Principle

The kinetic link principle provides both the framework for understanding and analyzing human movement patterns and the rationale for the use of exercise conditioning and rehabilitation programs that emphasize the entire body. Understanding the kinetic link principle highlights many of the concepts discussed in this book, particularly the integration of open and closed kinetic chain exercise.

Definition

The kinetic link principle describes how the human body can be considered as a series of interrelated links or segments. Movement of one segment affects segments both proximal and distal to the first segment. Kibler (1998a, 1998b) refers to the kinetic link system as a series of sequentially activated body segments. The kinetic link principle is predicated on a concept developed and described initially by Hanavan (1964), who constructed a computerized form of the adult human body. This computerized form comprises conical links that include the lower extremities, torso, and upper extremities. The forces generated by skill performance of upper-extremity segments are transmitted to the trunk and spine via a large musculoskeletal surface. This exchange of forces results in the generation of massive amounts of energy (Hanavan 1964).

Davies (1992) described how the upper extremity can be viewed as a series of links. The links proposed by Davies (1992) include the trunk, scapulothoracic articulation, scapulohumeral or glenohumeral joints, and distal arm regions. Each of these links can be considered independent anatomically and biomechanically, but with reference to human function must be considered as a unit.

Similar to the descriptions of the kinetic link by Hanavan (1964) and Davies (1992), Putnam (1993) has described the concept of proximal to distal sequencing. Used in the biomechanical analysis of human movement, the proximal to distal sequencing model also has relevance in exercise both for rehabilitation and performance enhancement. The terms kinetic link, proximal to distal sequencing, summation of speed principle (Bunn 1972), and Plagenhoef's (1971) concept of acceleration–deceleration all attempt to describe the complex interaction of the body's independent segments working together to form a functional unit or sequence of segments.

The goal of nearly all sport-related activities such as throwing, serving, and kicking a ball is to achieve maximal acceleration and hence the largest possible speed at the end of the linked segments (Bunn 1972). The concept states that motion ideally should be initiated with the more proximal segments and proceed to the more distal segments, with the more distal segment initiating its motion at the time of the maximal speed of the proximal segment. Each succeeding segment would generate larger end-point speeds than the proximal segment. This proximal to distal sequencing has been demonstrated in research by examining the linear speeds of segment end points, joint angular velocities, and resultant joint moments (Marshall and Elliott 2000).

Several investigators have demonstrated the proper proximal to distal sequencing in kicking (Marshall and Wood 1986; Putnam 1993). The linear speeds in the lower extremity when kicking a ball in the sagittal plane follow the proximal to distal sequence: The hip, knee, and ankle joints all reach their peak speeds in sequence, and each peak is greater than that of the proximal joint. Putnam (1993) felt that deceleration of the proximal segment occurs secondary to the acceleration of the distal segment. Other researchers (Marshall and Wood 1986) showed a reversal of the proximal joint torques late in the motion, which apparently serves to increase the speed of the distal segment.

Proximal to distal sequencing has been clearly identified in the tennis serve (Elliott et al. 1995; Groppel 1992; Plagenhoef 1971; VanGheluwe and Hebbelinck 1985) and throwing motion (Feltner and Dapena 1986). The literature in upper-extremity throwing or striking sports shows a modification of the proximal to distal pattern when the human body exploits the benefits of long-axis rotation of the humerus (internal rotation) and forearm (forearm pronation) to maximize end-point speed (Marshall and Elliott 2000). Research has demonstrated consistently that peak internal rotation of the shoulder (humerus) follows the movement of the wrist and hand (Elliott et al. 1995; Marshall and Elliott 2000; VanGheluwe and Hebbelinck 1985). Additionally, the peak speed of pronation has been found to occur immediately before ball contact on the tennis serve and forehand ground stroke, suggesting that this long-axis rotation does not conform to traditional explanations of proximal to distal sequencing (Marshall and Elliott 2000).

Groppel (1992) applied the kinetic link system to the analysis and description of optimal upper-extremity sport biomechanics. Groppel stated that the initiation of the sequential activation of the kinetic link system starts at the ground as the lower extremities create a ground reaction force. The sequential activation then proceeds from the legs, through the hips and trunk, and is funneled via the scapulothoracic and glenohumeral joints to the distal aspect of the upper extremity. Figure 3.1 shows the kinetic link system described by Groppel (1992). The important role of both linear and angular momentum in the production of force and power in upper-extremity sport activities such as the throwing motion and tennis serve is evident from an analysis of this model. It is important to note that initiation of movement of the next segment in the kinetic chain occurs before complete deceleration of the previous segment. The angular velocity of the segmental rotation in the body's kinetic link system was originally thought to occur at increasingly faster velocities from the lower to the upper extremities during the tennis serve (Groppel 1992). Further biomechanical analysis, as discussed earlier, has demonstrated that while this sequential increase in angular velocities does occur over many of the segments, a perfect progression in angular velocity does not occur (Elliott et al. 1986, Marshall and Elliott 2000).

Kibler (1994) provided an objective analysis of force generation during a tennis serve (table 3.1). Fifty-four percent of the force development during the tennis serve comes from the legs and trunk, with only 25% coming from the elbow and wrist. Nonoptimal performance and increased risk of injury occur in tennis and other sport activities when an individual attempts to use the smaller muscles and distal arm segments as a primary source for power generation (Groppel 1992; Kibler 1994).

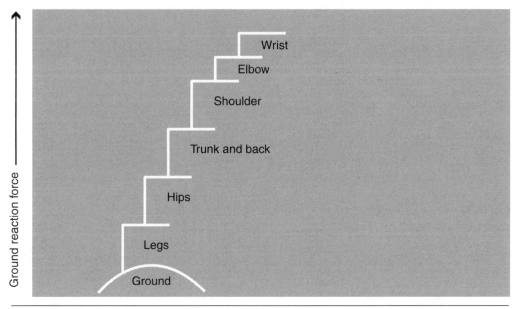

Figure 3.1   Kinetic link system.

Adapted from Groppel 1992.

Table 3.1   Specific Segments' Contribution to Kinetic Energy and Force Production in the Tennis Serve

Segment	Velocity (m/s)	Kinetic energy [units, (%)]	Force [units, (%)]
Leg/trunk	2.7	197.1 (51%)	729 (54%)
Shoulder	2.2	49.1 (13%)	297 (21%)
Elbow	6.4	82 (21%)	212 (15%)
Wrist	7.8	61 (15%)	130 (10%)

Adapted from Kibler 1994.

Use of the kinetic link principle is important when analyzing sport performance or exercise movement patterns. Movement patterns that do not sequentially activate all portions of the kinetic link system or that leave out a portion or link such as trunk rotation can lead to injury and nonoptimal performance (Groppel 1992; Kibler 1994). Examples of nonoptimal use of the kinetic link principle are depicted in figures 3.2 and 3.3. Figure 3.2 represents a missing segment from the normal sequential activation pattern, and figure 3.3 demonstrates improper timing of the sequential activation. These two examples are commonly encountered by the clinician when analyzing complex human movement patterns such as the tennis serve and throwing motion. It is very common for an individual to perform an activity without hip rotation because of either

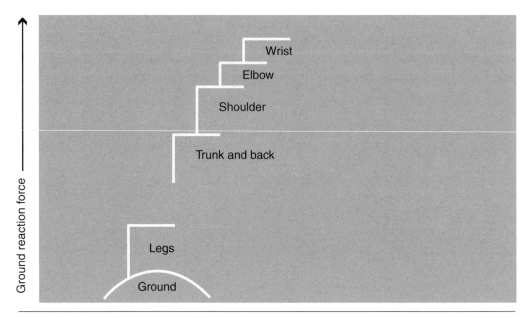

Figure 3.2 Nonoptimal use of the kinetic link system because of missing link.

Adapted from Groppel 1992.

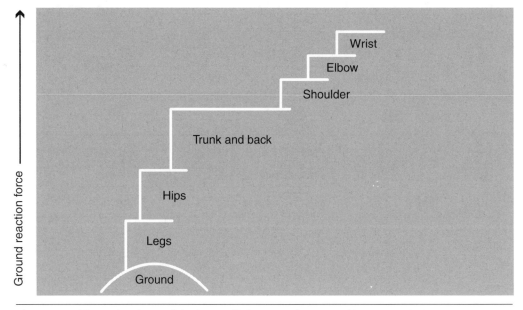

Figure 3.3 Nonoptimal use of the kinetic link system because of improper timing.

Adapted from Groppel 1992.

improper foot positioning or from inflexibility in the hip region. Additionally, inappropriate timing of trunk rotation can lead to disastrous consequences in segments proximal and distal to the trunk (Marshall et al. 1993).

A functional movement pattern such as the tennis serve would involve hitting the serve with little or no trunk rotation if the hips are precluded from rotating by an improper stance. This would produce greater loads and stresses to the shoulder and elbow and possibly result in injury. Additionally, if improper sequencing or timing of the rotation from the legs to the hip and trunk occurs, greater loads to the upper arm again are encountered. Marshall et al. (1993) used three-dimensional cinematography to analyze the mechanics of a highly skilled tennis player and the torques produced during the tennis serve. The effects on the medial aspect of the elbow of delaying internal shoulder rotation until late in the total movement were studied analytically. The amount of valgus stress to the medial elbow was increased 53% immediately before ball impact when nonoptimal timing was used during the serving motion. The effects of delaying internal shoulder rotation highlight the underlying concept behind the kinetic link principle during stressful upper-body sport movement.

Buckley and Kerwin (1988) demonstrated, again using the tennis serve, another important example of how the kinetic link system of the human body is applied during stressful musculoskeletal exertion. Elbow-extension velocities during the tennis serve were measured in elite tennis players and found to average 44 rad/s (2,521°/s). Upon initial analysis, many researchers and clinicians would assume that the triceps (elbow extensor) musculature was contracting concentrically to produce this elbow-extension velocity during the acceleration phase of the tennis serve. However, Jorgensen (1976) demonstrated that velocities beyond 20 rad/s (1,146°/s) are beyond the contractile velocity range of human skeletal muscle. Therefore, this finding can be explained by prior research by Quanbury et al. (1975) and Robertson and Winter (1980), which reported two sources of a limb's mechanical energy. The first, and most obvious, source is the muscles that are attached directly to the limb in question, and the second source is energy that flows passively across a joint from an adjoining limb. Therefore, the high resultant elbow-extension velocities measured during the tennis serve are not solely from the concentric triceps contraction, but also from the transfer of force from the proximal segments such as the trunk, scapula, and shoulder. These studies demonstrate the importance of the kinetic link system in human movement and also of training the entire limb or entire kinetic link of the body when attempting to affect a specific segment or link in the kinetic link system.

Total Arm Strength

Clinical and rehabilitative applications of the kinetic link system have led to the development of the concept of total arm strength (TAS) (Davies and Ellenbecker 1993). This concept is predicated on the kinetic link system and demonstrated by the close clinical relationship between shoulder and elbow injuries in sport. Priest and Nagel (1976) studied 84 world-class tennis players and reported that 74% of men and 60% of women had a history of shoulder or elbow injury in the dominant arm that affected tennis play. Injuries to both the shoulder and elbow of the dominant arm were reported by 21% and 23% of the men and women, respectively. Another study by Priest et al. (1980) surveyed 2,633 recreational tennis players and found an incidence of tennis elbow of 31%. Additionally there was a

Total arm strength principle is a rehabilitation concept that utilizes the kinetic link principle whereby strengthening of the entire extremity is carried out rather than merely isolating the injured segment.

63% greater incidence of shoulder injury among players who had a history of tennis elbow than among players who did not.

Another study of the total arm strength concept by Strizak et al. (1983) incorporated the isometric strength of the forearm (pronation and supination), wrist (radial and ulnar deviation, flexion and extension), and metacarpal phalangeal (MCP) joints (flexion and extension) to create a total arm strength index. This index was compared among three groups: (1) a normal, uninjured, non-tennis-playing control population, (2) healthy recreational tennis players, and (3) recreational tennis players with tennis elbow. Results of this study showed significantly greater total dominant arm strength relative to body weight in the control group and tennis-playing group, but no significant difference in the tennis elbow study population. The finding of greater total arm strength in both the control population and healthy tennis players but not in the injured group supports the use of whole-extremity, or in this application total arm strength, rehabilitation and conditioning programs.

Total Leg Strength

The concept of total arm strength is paralleled in the lower extremity by the concept of total leg strength (TLS). Nicholas et al. (1976) isokinetically tested the hip flexors, abductors, adductors, quadriceps, and hamstrings and added all those individual strength measures together to create a TLS parameter. They found proximal muscular weakness in the lower extremities with plantarflexion/inversion ankle sprains. Gleim et al. (1978) expanded on the original work of Nicholas et al. (1976) by correlating individual muscle deficits and TLS deficits with injuries in 219 patients. Their research established that a 10% isolated muscular deficit significantly correlated to lower-extremity injury. Of particular interest was the finding that a 5% deficit in the TLS parameter significantly correlated to lower-extremity injury.

Additionally, Bullock-Saxton (1994) found local sensation changes and an alteration of proximal (gluteus maximus) hip muscle function in subjects following severe ankle sprains. Bolz and Davies (1984) tested isokinetic hip extension and flexion, abduction and adduction, knee extension and flexion, and ankle plantar flexion and dorsiflexion in 24 subjects. They found significant unilateral muscular weakness in the TLS factor (summing all measures from the eight motions tested) in 8 out of the 24 subjects who had a leg length discrepancy of 0.5 cm or more. The TLS factor revealed a consistent weakness in the short leg in these subjects.

Summary

This chapter summarized some of the relevant anatomical and biomechanical relationships in the kinetic link system of the human body. This chapter also pointed out the potential benefits of exercises that work multiple joints and muscle groups and stress and challenge the body's kinetic link system. Integration of the kinetic link system and the concepts of total arm and total leg strength presented in this chapter will provide the clinician with a functionally specific framework that can lead to optimal program design for both performance enhancement and injury rehabilitation. The following chapters focus on the application of closed kinetic chain exercises to address the body as a series of links, based on the important concepts detailed in this chapter.

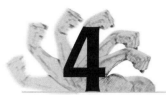

4

Comparison of Open and Closed Kinetic Chain Exercise

This chapter emphasizes the need for critical thinking about the appropriate functional applications of open and closed kinetic chain exercises in rehabilitation and orthopedics. Both types of exercises have their indications, contraindications, and applications in the testing and rehabilitation of various pathological conditions. The purposes of this chapter are

- to separate fact from fiction regarding the benefits of closed kinetic chain exercise,
- to review the characteristics of open and closed kinetic chain exercises, and
- to provide a functional testing algorithm for the appropriate selection and implementation of these exercises.

The Scientific Basis for Exercise Selection

Open kinetic chain and closed kinetic chain exercises have been used for many years in rehabilitation. However, the use of these various exercises has varied considerably over time. For example, over the last 30 years, the trends in the use of these exercises were generally as listed directly below. The predicted trend for the 2000s is the integration of open and closed kinetic chain functional rehabilitation.

1970s	Functional rehabilitation
1980s	Open kinetic chain exercises (with emphasis on isokinetics)
1990s	Closed kinetic chain exercises

There are several prevalent theories about closed kinetic chain exercises that explain why they were the preferred mode of the 1990s. The theories emphasize that closed kinetic chain exercises are functional, create a co-contraction of the quadriceps and hamstrings, and cause less stress to the anterior cruciate ligament (ACL) graft in cases of ACL reconstruction. Davies (1995b) recommended that readers use critical thinking in the analysis and application of what exercises they use and to consider the published scientific rationale behind the choices of the various exercises.

Functionality

There are several reasons that clinicians use closed kinetic chain exercise and de-emphasize open kinetic chain exercise. One of the common arguments against the primary use of open kinetic chain exercises in the lower extremity is that they are not functional. For example, there are limited instances where an individual functions in a seated position bending and straightening the leg. Therefore, the knee-extension exercise is often seen as nonfunctional rather than a functional rehabilitation activity. Closed kinetic chain exercises are considered to be more functional, particularly in the lower extremity, because they closely simulate the actual movement patterns encountered in both sport and daily activities.

Analysis of most functional activities reveals that they are, in fact, a series of successive open kinetic chain and closed kinetic chain motions. An example is the normal gait cycle. During walking, approximately 65% of the gait cycle is weight bearing (closed kinetic chain) and 35% is non–weight bearing (open kinetic chain). Interestingly, during running, the percentages of closed and open kinetic chain motions essentially reverse. During sprinting, the percentages change even more dramatically: Only about 5% to 10% of the cycle is closed kinetic chain, and 90% to 95% is open kinetic chain. This illustration demonstrates that functional activities are not just closed kinetic chain motions, but a combination of both open and closed (Wilk et al. 1995). Most injuries that occur to the lower extremity, such as ankle sprains and contact and noncontact ACL injuries, usually occur in the closed kinetic chain position. However, little scientific evidence supports the theory that doing only closed kinetic chain exercises can prevent these injuries.

A few studies show minimal correlation between closed kinetic chain and open kinetic chain tests (Andersen et al. 1995; Delitto et al. 1993; Feiring and Ellenbecker 1996; Greenberger and Paterno 1995; Swarup et al. 1992). However, more studies demonstrate a correlation between closed kinetic chain and open kinetic chain tests and a correlation to functional performance (Anderson 1989; Anderson et al. 1991; Barber et al. 1990; Noyes et al. 1991; Sachs et al. 1989; Schaffer et al. 1994; Tegner et al. 1986; Wiklander and Lysholm 1987; Wilk et al. 1994). Therefore, assuming that open kinetic chain testing and training are not functional is not supported in the literature. Even though the open kinetic chain movement pattern is not always a functional movement pattern in and of itself, it does correlate with functional tests and can be integrated into most functional rehabilitation programs.

Co-Contraction

Many clinicians have assumed that in the closed kinetic chain position of the lower extremity there is automatically a resultant co-contraction of the muscles that should dynamically stabilize the knee joint. Although some studies (Johansson et al. 1989; Renstrom et al. 1986) did demonstrate this phenomenon, several recent studies (Escamilla et al. 1998; Isear et al. 1997) actually refuted that significant co-contractions occur with some closed kinetic chain exercises.

Anterior Cruciate Ligament Strain

Another widely held belief is that less strain occurs in the ACL with closed than with open kinetic chain exercise regimens. Consequently, it is common clinical practice to initiate exercises that require the foot to be fixed against resistance in the initial stages of ACL rehabilitation (Silfverskiold et al. 1988). Only after adequate ACL graft healing occurs does the individual progress to open kinetic chain exercises in the non-weight-bearing knee. The theories supporting this approach are that closed kinetic chain (weight-bearing) exercises result in less anterior–posterior displacement of the tibia on the femur because of co-contraction of the leg muscles spanning the joint and because of the compressive joint loads produced by body weight forcing the articular surfaces together. As previously stated, the validity of co-contraction must be reevaluated. Multiple studies using cadaveric models (Hsieh and Walker 1976; More et al. 1993), electromyographic activity monitoring (Ohkoshi et al. 1991), mathematical models (Lutz et al. 1993), and instrumented knee-laxity devices (Lysholm and Messner 1995; Yack et al. 1993) indirectly suggested that less force is placed through the ACL during closed kinetic chain exercise, but they provided mostly indirect evidence of this.

In a landmark study, Beynnon et al. (1997) directly measured in vivo ACL strain by implanting a differential variable reluctance transducer (DVRT) on the ACL of subjects who performed closed kinetic chain and open kinetic chain exercises with normal muscle function and joint loading. The subjects performed the following activities: (1) open kinetic chain knee flexion to extension from $0°$ to $100°$, (2) closed kinetic chain squats from $0°$ to $100°$, and (3) closed kinetic chain squats from $0°$ to $100°$ with sport-cord resistance with a load sensor. Although these authors' original hypothesis was in keeping with popular theories and some prior research, the results showed no significant difference in average maximal ACL strain values produced by open kinetic chain active flexion–extension (3.5%), closed kinetic chain squatting (3.6%), and closed kinetic chain resisted squatting (4.0%). In each exercise, the maximal ACL strain occurred at extension and decreased progressively as the knee was flexed to $100°$. Additionally, there was no significant difference in maximal ACL strain values among these exercises at $10°$, $20°$, and $90°$. The findings of this study are a departure from previous clinical studies and accepted theory concerning ACL rehabilitation. The authors speculated that it may not be valid to designate closed kinetic chain or open kinetic chain activities as "safe" and "unsafe" for rehabilitation of the injured ACL or healing graft.

Another interesting interpretation of research comparing closed kinetic chain and open kinetic chain exercises is in a study by Bynum et al. (1995). This was one of the first prospective randomized studies comparing open and closed kinetic chain exercises. This study reached the following conclusions about the closed kinetic chain training group:

1. Lower mean KT1000 Arthrometer side-to-side differences (20 lb: $p = .057$, not significant; manual maximum: $p = .018$, significant)

2. Less patellofemoral pain ($p = .48$, not significant)

3. Generally more satisfied with the end result ($p = .36$, not significant)

4. Returned to activities of daily living (ADLs) sooner than expected ($p = .007$, significant)

5. Returned to sports sooner than expected ($p = .118$, not significant)

Bynum et al. (1995) stated: "As a result of this study, we now use the closed kinetic chain protocol exclusively after anterior cruciate ligament reconstruction." Surprisingly, these researchers deduced several conclusions that were not statistically or clinically significant, yet they based their entire protocol exclusively on these findings.

Snyder-Mackler (1996) described the common approach to many rehabilitation programs in the following manner:

> Rehabilitation after reconstruction of the anterior cruciate ligament continues to be guided more by myth and fad than by science. Intensive closed kinetic chain exercise has virtually replaced open kinetic chain exercise of the quadriceps after a reconstruction. . . . The present study confirms the finding that strength of the quadriceps femoris has a substantial impact on functional recovery and suggests that closed kinetic chain exercise alone does *not* provide an adequate stimulus to the quadriceps femoris to permit more normal function of the knee in stance phase in most patients in the early period after reconstruction of the anterior cruciate ligament. . . . We believe that the judicious application of open kinetic chain exercises for the quadriceps femoris muscle (with the knee in a position that does not stress the graft) improves the strength of this muscle and functional outcome after reconstruction of the anterior cruciate ligament.

The balance of this chapter emphasizes the need for critical thinking (Davies 1995b) regarding the appropriate functional applications of open and closed kinetic chain exercises in rehabilitation.

Characteristics of Open and Closed Kinetic Chain Exercise

There are probably few activities that can be classified as purely open kinetic chain or closed kinetic chain activities; most activities exist along a continuum incorporating components of both. An illustration of an open kinetic chain activity is a seated knee flexion-to-extension movement. There are several characteristics that describe this pattern of movement, but a key quality is that the distal end of the extremity is free in space, not fixed to anything, and does not bear weight. This seated knee flexion-to-extension pattern serves as a model to demonstrate the characteristics of open kinetic chain exercises. The characteristics in table 4.1 are often used to describe open kinetic chain exercises (Davies 1995a; Davies, Heiderscheit, Clark 2000; Fitzgerald 1997; Freidhoff et al. 1998; Rivera 1994; Wilk et al. 1995; Wilk, Escamilla et al. 1996; Yack et al. 1993).

Activities progress along a continuum from closed to open kinetic chain, with many activities of daily living and sport activities incorporating components of both. For example, during the gait cycle, the stance phase is a closed kinetic chain pattern, whereas the swing phase is an open kinetic chain pattern. Another example that shows the interplay between these two movement patterns is riding a bike, during which the foot is fixed on the pedal in a closed kinetic chain pattern, yet the pedal and foot freely move in space. Another example is skiing, where the feet are fixed to the skis (closed kinetic chain), but the skis move on the snow and are not fixed to an object (open kinetic chain).

A classification system that tries to incorporate this continuum was described by Wilk et al. (1995). In this classification, exercises or activities progress from open kinetic chain succession drills to partial kinetic chain–closed kinetic chain activities. This classification attempts to describe exercises that often do not fit cleanly into the traditional open and closed kinetic chain classification presented in chapter 1. Succession drills and partial kinetic chain activities are terms used to describe these activities (Wilk et al. 1995).

When the distal end of the extremity is fixed to something, typically in a weight-bearing position, the exercise or activity becomes a closed kinetic chain activity. The squat maneuver can be used as a model to illustrate this closed kinetic chain pattern. The characteristics listed in table 4.2 are often used to describe closed

Table 4.1 Characteristics of Open Kinetic Chain Exercise

Distal end of the extremity is free in space.

Distal end of the extremity is not in contact with a fixed object.

Movement pattern is characterized by rotary stress in the joint.

Joint movements occur in isolation.

Muscle recruitment and movements are isolated.

Joint axis is stable during movement patterns.

The proximal segment that forms the joint is stable, and the distal segment is mobile.

Motion occurs distal to the instantaneous axis of rotation.

Movement pattern is often nonfunctional.

Movement causes shear forces in the joint.

Artificial loading of the muscles and joints occurs.

Velocity is predetermined by exercise equipment if isokinetics is used.

There is an artificial means of stabilization.

Testing is not typically functional.

Table 4.2 Characteristics of Closed Kinetic Chain Exercise

Distal end of the extremity is fixed to something.

Movement pattern is characterized by linear stress in the joint.

Multiple joint movements occur simultaneously.

Multiple muscles are recruited.

The primary joint axis is transverse.

Both segments that form the joint move simultaneously.

Movement patterns are functional.

Movement causes compressive forces in a joint.

There is co-contraction of the muscles surrounding the joint.

Movement often occurs in multiple planes simultaneously.

Muscles and joints are physiologically loaded.

Velocity is variable through a movement pattern.

There is no artificial stabilization.

Loading is physiological and provides normal proprioceptive or kinesthetic feedback.

Performance of movement is not inhibited by design of equipment.

Movement causes compression of the joint surfaces, thereby increasing joint stability.

Testing and exercises are more functional.

kinetic chain exercises (Davies et al. 1995; Davies, Heiderscheit, Clark 2000; Fitzgerald 1997; Freidhoff et al. 1998; Rivera 1994; Wilk et al. 1995; Wilk, Escamilla, et al. 1996; Yack et al. 1993).

Although many of the characteristics in tables 4.1 and 4.2 have been used to describe open and closed kinetic chain exercises, the more important question is, "Why would we want to use each type of exercise in testing and rehabilitation?" The following section describes the rationale for performing the respective types of exercises in orthopedic testing and rehabilitation.

Functional Testing Algorithm for Open and Closed Kinetic Chain Activities

An **algorithm** is a specific, organized method for problem solving.

A systematic evaluation process is important for the clinician to make the appropriate selection of exercises to use in a functional rehabilitation program. This section describes a functional testing algorithm (FTA) that the authors of this book have used for many years in the clinical setting (Davies 1995a; Davies and Ellenbecker 1998; Davies, Heiderscheit, and Clark 2000; Davies, Wilk, and Ellenbecker 1997). This FTA is an objective, quantitative, and systematic testing and rehabilitation strategy intended to progress a patient safely and rapidly to full functional activity after an injury or surgery. The progression from one stage to the next stage in the FTA is based on the patient passing the prior test in a series of sequential tests. Each successive test and its associated training regimen places increased stress on the injured part while decreasing clinical control.

Established criteria must be met for the patient to progress through the FTA. The criteria are based on published research, years of clinical experience, and empirically based clinical guidelines. These criteria are summarized in table 4.3.

Functional Testing Algorithm Protocol

The FTA consists of basic tests and measurements, strength and power testing, and functional testing. Figure 4.1 summarizes the entire FTA. The following

Table 4.3 Empirical Guidelines for Patient Progression in the Functional Testing Algorithm

Test	Empirical guidelines
Subjective	Pain < 3 (analog pain scale: 0–10)
Basic measurements	< 10% difference in bilateral comparison
KT1000	< 3 mm difference in bilateral comparison
Digital balance evaluation (DBE)	< 30% bilateral comparison
Closed kinetic chain (CKC), supine	< 30% difference in bilateral comparison
Open kinetic chain (OKC)	< 25% difference in bilateral comparison
Closed kinetic chain (CKC), standing	< 20% difference in bilateral comparison
Functional jump test (FJT)	≥ 80% of body height and norms
Functional hop test (FHT)	< 15% difference in bilateral comparison and norms
Lower-extremity functional test (LEFT)	Female < 2 min; male < 1.5 min
Sport-specific testing (SST)	

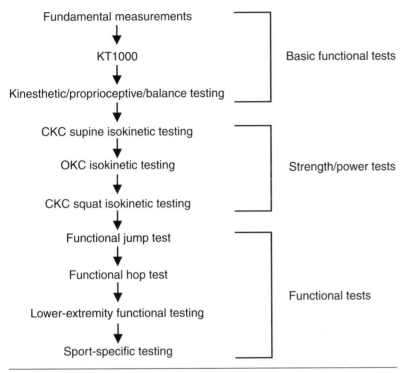

Figure 4.1   Functional testing algorithm for the lower extremity.

sections briefly describe the steps in this process. The results of the tests dictate the types of exercises that a patient will perform during the rehabilitation program. Because of the common incidence of knee injuries and the widespread use of closed and open kinetic chain exercises in testing and rehabilitation of various knee conditions, the knee serves as the model for this discussion.

Fundamental Measurements

The fundamental measurements include pain graded on a visual analog scale (VAS), anthropometric measurements, and goniometric measurements. Once most of these variables have normalized during the rehabilitation program (measurements on both injured and uninjured within 10% of each other or within normal limits of descriptive normative data) then the patient advances in the FTA.

Muscular Strength and Power Testing

Muscular strength and power form the core of most functional activities. Open and closed kinetic chain tests are used to assess muscular strength and power in the FTA.

Closed Kinetic Chain Isokinetic Testing: Semisitting or Supine Position

Because of the increased emphasis over the last decade on closed kinetic chain exercises as functional exercises, it is important to measure closed kinetic chain performance. Because closed kinetic chain exercises are supposed to be safer for the knee because they are functional, increase joint compressive forces, promote co-contractions of the quadriceps and hamstring muscles, and minimize translatory stresses to the ligaments, closed kinetic chain testing is performed first.

Anthropometric measurements are circumferential measurements taken at various points along a limb to determine muscular girth (atrophy or hypertrophy) as well as swelling.

Testing in the closed kinetic chain position is initially performed using a Linea computerized isokinetic/isotonic testing and rehabilitation system. Davies and Heiderscheit (1997) published results on the reliability of the Linea. Their study demonstrated that the intraclass correlation coefficients vary from .85 to .94, which is a good to excellent test-retest reliability. The FTA evaluates the patient's performance on this test using the criteria established in table 4.3, allowing the clinician to make a decision regarding the patient's status. If the patient passes the test, then he or she progresses to the next higher level of the FTA. If the patient fails the minimally established criteria, then the patient's rehabilitation program focuses on rehabilitation techniques or exercises that are designed to help the patient improve the specific deficit. Examples of specific closed kinetic chain and open kinetic chain exercises for rehabilitation or performance-enhancement programs are described later in this book. Examples of specific relative contraindications for closed kinetic chain testing of the knee are mild pain, mild effusion, limited range of motion, and recency of injury or surgery.

Open Kinetic Chain Testing

The next stage of the FTA is to perform open kinetic chain testing of the specific muscle groups that are targeted for rehabilitation based on the examination findings. With any condition and with any type of testing, there are always relative and absolute contraindications for testing. Examples of specific relative contraindications for open kinetic chain testing of the knee are mild pain, mild effusion, limited range of motion, and recency of injury or surgery. Absolute contraindications are significant pain, major effusion, major range of motion limitations, acute condition, patellofemoral chondrosis, tendinitis (leading to pain with exertion), and insufficient healing time following an injury or surgery.

There are many reasons for performing open kinetic chain testing to evaluate the status of the patient's present condition:

- To assess whether or not there are any isolated muscular deficits (Davies 1992; Nicholas et al. 1976; Snyder-Mackler 1996). If a muscle cannot function normally in an isolated manner (open kinetic chain), then it cannot function normally in a functional (closed kinetic chain) pattern.
- To evaluate the individual parts of the total leg strength (Gleim et al. 1978; Snyder-Mackler 1996).
- To sample a muscle's ability at different speeds using velocity spectrum testing (Davies 1992).
- To identify the weak link in the kinetic chain, that is, the link where neuromuscular timing and recruitment of the muscles are impaired (Davies 1992).

Open kinetic chain testing has inherent clinical controls that make it safe:

- No varus, valgus, or rotation during the testing (Davies et al. 1995)
- A proximally placed tibial pad that helps reduce anterior translation of the tibia (Davies 1995a; Wilk and Andrews 1993; Wilk et al. 1994)
- Controlled speeds that can minimize anterior translation (Davies et al. 1995; Wilk and Andrews 1993; Wilk et al. 1994)
- Precise control of range of motion

The authors of this book perform isokinetic open kinetic chain testing to get an objective number for the specific performance of individual muscles as separate components of the entire kinetic chain.

Data calculation involves evaluating various parameters from the computerized testing, such as peak torque, total work, average power, and torque acceleration energy. The data need to be further evaluated by analyzing bilateral comparisons, unilateral ratios of agonist to antagonist muscle groups, peak torque to body weight, and so on to customize the rehabilitation program for the patient.

If the patient meets the minimum criteria in this category, he or she progresses to the next stage of the FTA. If the patient demonstrates significant deficits during this test, then the focus of the rehabilitation program is on this particular limitation, along with other components of the rehabilitation or performance-enhancement program.

Closed Kinetic Chain Weight-Bearing Squat Isokinetic Testing

The next test in the strength and power sequence is in a closed kinetic chain weight-bearing squat position. The Linea is placed in the upright position, and the testing is performed in the weight-bearing position. The same format is applied: The patient either progresses to the next level of the FTA or focuses his or her rehabilitation program on the particular deficits found with this testing.

Functional Testing

The essential element of any testing sequence must involve functional testing specific to the patient and his or her activities. A major change in the FTA at this stage is that there is no longer much clinical control imposed on the patient. All the advantages listed under open kinetic chain testing are now lost. Consequently, the lower extremity is subjected to increased varus or valgus and rotational stresses without any limitations or clinical control.

Functional Jump Test

The functional testing sequence begins with a two-legged functional jump test. This test measures the patient's functional bilateral lower-leg power. Therefore, to prevent segmental contributions from the arms, neck, and trunk, the patients grasp their hands behind their back to minimize compensatory movements (Davies and Zillmer 2000). The patient performs a series of four gradient submaximal to maximal warm-ups (25, 50, 75, 100%) and then performs three maximal test repetitions. In addition to giving a quantitative value for the patient's performance, this test assesses the patient's readiness to perform uncontrolled functional activities. The data analysis is performed by averaging three maximal volitional jumps and then normalizing the data to the patient's height, as summarized in table 4.4. If the patient meets the minimum criteria, he or she

Table 4.4   Functional (Relative/Normalized) Jump and Hop Test

	Males (distance as % of height)	Females (distance as % of height)
Jump test (R + L)	90–100	80–90
Hop test (uninjured leg)	80–90	70–80
Hop test (injured leg)	80–90	70–80

progresses to the next testing sequence in the FTA; otherwise, the rehabilitation program is designed to improve the patient's performance in this type of activity pattern.

Functional Hop Test

The functional hop test is a single-leg test in which the patient jumps and lands on the same extremity. This functional test is recommended by the International Knee Documentation Committee (IKDC). This is a significant progression from the two-legged jump test because now the patient must take off from (concentric movement pattern) and land (uncontrolled eccentric movement pattern) on the involved extremity. The authors of this book think that this is one of the most important tests to demonstrate the patient's psychological readiness to use and stress the involved extremity in a functional manner.

The testing format is similar to the jump testing, with a series of four gradient submaximal to maximal volitional effort tests. The test is evaluated by both the quantitative values and the qualitative performance. If the patient demonstrates any hesitation, limping, or significant abnormal angulation, it indicates that deficits are still present and need to be addressed in the rehabilitation program.

The bilateral data are compared (IKDC reports that bilateral results within 10% to 15% are excellent) and normalized to the patient's height, as indicated in table 4.4. The reason for the normalization is best demonstrated in this example. If a patient hops 43 inches (109 cm) on the right uninvolved leg and 40 inches (102 cm) on the left involved leg, then the values are within 10% of each other. However, this bilateral comparison does not take into account the competence of the uninjured extremity. If the patient's healthy limb's baseline performance is substandard, the assumption that the patient's injured extremity is fully rehabilitated because the injured leg's performance was within 10% of that of the uninjured extremity may be incorrect. To avoid such bad assumptions, a normalized parameter is achieved by dividing the actual performance distance by the patient's height to obtain a percentage. In this example, if the patient is 65 inches (165 cm) tall, he or she still has a residual deficit based on the normalized parameter.

Lower-Extremity Functional Test

When the patient reaches the final stages of the rehabilitation program and is being considered for discharge, it is time to perform a lower-extremity functional test (LEFT). This test, which the authors have used for many years, incorporates many functional movement patterns in a progressively stressful testing sequence (table 4.5). The configuration of the course and the sequence of the patterns in the LEFT are illustrated in figures 4.2 and 4.3.

A multicenter reliability test was performed on the LEFT, and the results were excellent. Tabor et al. (1999) tested 27 subjects in a test-retest paradigm with one week between the tests and found, using paired t tests ($p = .05$), that there was no difference between the test sessions. An intraclass correlation coefficient of .953 was determined. Therefore, the LEFT is a highly reliable functional test to demonstrate a patient's functional performance abilities.

Descriptive normative data that have been collected on thousands of subjects and patients over the years (from the authors' unpublished data) are described in table 4.6.

Table 4.5   Sequence of the LEFT

1. Forward run
2. Backward run
3. Side shuffles (both ways)
4. Cariocas (both ways)
5. Figure-eight run (both ways)
6. 45° angle cuts (outside foot, both ways)
7. 90° angle cuts (outside foot, both ways)
8. 90° crossover cuts (both ways)
9. Forward run
10. Backward run

Activity-Specific Testing

The final stage of the FTA is testing of the patient's final performance in specific activities such as ADLs, vocational activities, recreational activities, or competitive sports. This testing is individualized to the patient and is similar to an ergonomic test and then appropriate work hardening to actually prepare the patient to return to the particular activity.

Time Commitment for Testing

Often, when individuals read about this functional testing algorithm, they indicate that they do not have the time or resources for numbers of visits. Admittedly, testing and evaluating the patient's status does take time. However, knowing the precise status of the patient through testing actually saves time because treatments can be more focused rather than generalized.

The authors in their clinic have the equip-

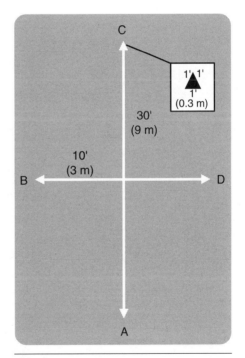

Figure 4.2 Configuration and dimensions of course for lower-extremity function test.

ment and resources to perform this type of testing, rehabilitation, and progression. One does not have to use this format, however, although some type of progressive evaluation and adjustments based on the exam findings should be used.

With managed care rather than outcomes research often driving treatment programs and deciding what is best for the patient, clinicians often comment, "Well, I only have so many visits with my patient." Clinicians who have limited visits with their patients should test and treat, rather than just treat the patient. If the patient is tested, the clinician knows the patient's precise status. This allows for customization of the rehabilitation and home exercise program based on the patient's needs. Therefore, the use of the FTA allows the clinician to be even more efficient with the limited number of patient visits available. The philosophy "If I

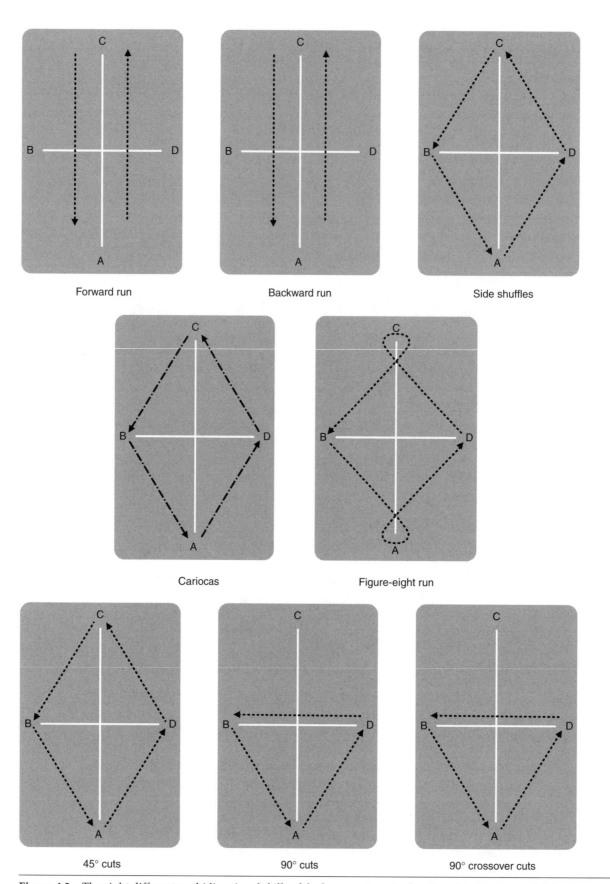

Figure 4.3 The eight different multidirectional skills of the lower-extremity functional test in the established sequence.

Table 4.6   Lower-Extremity Functional Test Descriptive Normative Data

Norms					
Males			Females		
90 s	l00 s*	125 s	120 s	135 s*	150 s

* Average.

treat you today, I help you today" is shortsighted. The philosophy "If I test you, treat you, and teach you a home exercise program, I will help you for a lifetime" is more efficacious.

Summary

The scientific and clinical rationale for using both open and closed kinetic chain exercises was described in this chapter, and their characteristics were reviewed. A systematic functional testing algorithm for rehabilitation was also presented. This chapter provided the background information needed to integrate both open and closed kinetic chain exercise and testing techniques. The next chapters provide more specific applications for both the upper and lower extremity.

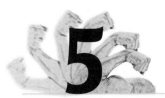

5

Closed Kinetic Chain Exercise for Rehabilitation and Conditioning of the Lower Extremity

Most of the activities of the lower extremity occur in what has traditionally been described as a closed kinetic chain environment. Lower-extremity movement patterns range from ambulation, where the angular velocities of the knee range from approximately 200°/s, to running, with angular velocities over 1,000°/s. However, even though much emphasis is placed on closed kinetic chain exercises being functional, it is important to remember that most functional activities are really combinations of alternating closed and open kinetic chain activities. Because of the integrated movement patterns associated with most human motions of the lower extremities, a multimodal testing and training program is recommended for rehabilitation and performance enhancement. Specificity for performance activities should dictate the type of testing and training used.

Lower-Extremity Closed Kinetic Chain Training

Several studies have been conducted that demonstrate the efficacy of closed kinetic chain training. Worrell et al. (1993) conducted a four-week closed chain step-up training program using healthy subjects. They found significant improvement in closed chain leg press, step-up, and hop for both distance and time. No significant improvement was measured in open chain isokinetic knee-extension strength following training using an 8-inch (20 cm) step closed kinetic chain exercise program.

In a similar study, Koenig et al. (1995) studied subjects during a 10-week bench-step aerobics program. A group of novice steppers performed 50 minutes of stepping three times a week for 10 weeks using only body-weight resistance. No significant isolated quadriceps or hamstring strength improvements were found using isokinetic open chain testing. Stiene et al. (1996) compared the effects of eight weeks of either open or closed kinetic chain training in patients with patellofemoral pain. Isokinetic knee extension and an 8-inch (20 cm) step test were used to measure strength in the open and closed kinetic chain, respectively. In contrast to the studies presented earlier in this section, Stiene et al. (1996) found improvements in isokinetic thigh strength in both the open and closed kinetic chain training groups, but improvement in closed chain testing (8-inch step test) and functional status via a subjective questionnaire was greater in the closed kinetic chain training group. These studies suggest specific training and testing adaptations from open and closed kinetic chain training and the need for the integration of closed chain training with other modes of exercise training to ensure a complete and functional training stimulus.

In addition to research using step-up training, several studies have examined the use of leg-press and squat training. Augustsson et al. (1998) compared six weeks of knee-extension and hip-adduction open chain training to six weeks' training using a barbell squat. Significant improvements in closed chain squat performance were noted in both groups after six weeks of training, although the closed chain training group improved more than the open chain training group. No improvements were measured in open chain isokinetic knee-extension strength in either group; only the closed chain training group demonstrated improvements in a vertical jump test. Specificity of training again appears to be an important factor in producing changes in lower-extremity muscular strength and function.

Wawrzyniak et al. (1996) studied the effects of six weeks of unilateral leg-press training in nonathletic college women. Closed chain training using a leg-press motion resulted in significant isokinetic quadriceps strength improvement both concentrically and eccentrically, as well as improvements in a hop test for distance. This study showed a significant carryover from closed chain training using a unilateral leg press to quadriceps strength measured using an isolated open kinetic chain knee-extension test.

Loy et al. (1994) studied the effects of stair climbing on quadriceps strength. Subjects performed 12 weeks of stair climbing with no load and with loads of 4% and 8% of body weight. Significant improvements were measured in isokinetic peak torque and total work of the quadriceps for the subjects who trained with and without an external load. These authors concluded that a closed chain stair-climbing exercise results in improvements in quadriceps strength following 12 weeks of training.

Feiring and Ellenbecker (1996) tested 23 patients, 15 weeks following ACL reconstruction with an autogenous patellar tendon graft, using both an isokinetic open kinetic chain knee-extension test and an isokinetic closed chain leg-press test. Results showed a return of closed chain isokinetic leg-press extension strength to 91° to 93% of the contralateral side. Open kinetic chain knee-extension isokinetic strength was only 74° to 77% of the contralateral side, demonstrating a tremendous difference in the measurement of lower-extremity strength between the open and closed kinetic chain. The differences in lower-extremity strength measured in this study clearly demonstrate the role specificity plays in training and testing, and is an additional issue that must be considered in the utilization of testing and training techniques for the musculoskeletal system. Careful monitoring of both isolated open kinetic chain muscular strength as well as closed chain multiple-joint performance is indicated based on the results of this and other studies.

Davies (1995a) tested 200 patients with various knee injuries and found similar results to the Feiring and Ellenbecker (1996) research. The closed kinetic chain extension testing showed an average deficit of 10% when compared to the uninjured contralateral extremity whereas the open kinetic chain testing of the quadriceps was 25%. This study also demonstrates the need for assessment of both open and closed kinetic chain muscular strength and function following lower-extremity injury or during performance enhancement training.

These studies show some overflow, or carryover, between open and closed kinetic chain exercise modes, as well as specificity issues regarding closed kinetic chain training for the lower extremities. Further research is needed to more clearly understand the effects of many of the currently used closed chain training methods on isolated muscular strengthening and functional performance.

Overflow, often used interchangeably with carryover, is a term used to describe the persistence of a training response from a specific type of training to an additional parameter or variable that was not trained or specifically emphsized.

A recent study that took a novel approach to evaluating lower-extremity closed kinetic chain weight bearing was performed by Neitzel et al. (2000). Ninety-six subjects were monitored during execution of a parallel squat using a Smith squat rack and Pedar in-shoe force sensors to determine bilateral weight-bearing patterns during the exercise. Twenty-four subjects were sampled from each of four groups:

1. Patients 6 to 12 weeks after ACL reconstruction
2. Patients 6 to 7 months after ACL reconstruction
3. Patients 12 to 15 months after ACL reconstruction
4. Age-matched control group with no lower-extremity injury

Subjects in all groups performed three sets of nine squats to each of three flexion angles (30°, 60°, and 90°) and with three different weights (40-lb [18 kg] bar only, 35% body weight, and 50% body weight). Subjects were also asked if they felt that they had demonstrated weight bearing by both legs equally during the squat exercise.

Results of the study showed that healthy control-group subjects had equal bilateral weight bearing during execution of the squat during all conditions. In contrast, the patients between 6 and 12 weeks after ACL reconstruction "unloaded" the involved lower extremity during closed kinetic chain exercises at all three flexion angles. Six months after ACL reconstruction, subjects also unloaded the involved extremity in all three angular conditions. Finally, one year after ACL reconstruction, subjects demonstrated symmetrical weight-bearing patterns in their lower extremities similar to the control-group subjects.

The clinical significance of this study is that performing only closed kinetic chain exercises following ACL reconstruction may lead to unloading of the involved extremity for up to a year following surgery. Therefore, integration of single-leg closed kinetic chain exercises may be necessary to provide a more realistic and better level of stimulus to the recovering lower extremity. It is through clinical research such as this that clinicians can understand the rationale and receive guidance for the optimal progression and application of resistive exercise in rehabilitation and performance enhancement.

Integration of Closed Kinetic Chain Testing and Training

The use of closed kinetic chain testing and training is demonstrated by the Davies functional testing algorithm presented in chapter 4. Figure 5.1 includes the guidelines for patient progress through the rehabilitation program.

In this chapter, some specific closed kinetic chain training methods are covered, focusing on the elements that are determined to be deficient by applying the closed and open kinetic chain tests discussed in chapter 4.

Kinesthetic, Proprioceptive, and Balance Testing and Training

If the digital balance evaluation or other type of lower-extremity balance test determines that a kinesthetic, proprioceptive, or balance deficit exists, emphasis is placed on kinesthetic exercises for neuromuscular control. Examples of exercises that can be used in the rehabilitation program include biofeedback training in open and closed kinetic chain positions, co-contraction exercises, balance exercises progressing from stable to unstable training surfaces, double- to single-leg exercises, low-level functional exercises, and fundamental neuromuscular coordination drills. Virtually any closed kinetic chain training exercise can be adapted to increase the amount of kinesthetic and proprioceptive balance feedback to the body. Implements such as a balance board, half-cut foam rolls, foam pads and cushions, or even a standard bed pillow can create a more unstable surface for execution of closed kinetic chain exercises. See chapter 7 for examples of exercises to promote lower-extremity kinesthetic and proprioceptive function.

Perturbation training uses uneven or unstable supportive surfaces and forces and distractions to challenge the proprioceptive and kinesthetic systems of the body.

Fitzgerald et al. (2000) studied the effects of what they termed *perturbation training* in patients undergoing nonoperative rehabilitation following ACL injury. They compared two groups: one with traditional ACL rehabilitation and a group that received standard rehabilitation with the addition of perturbation training. The perturbation training involved closed kinetic chain exercises and postures using unstable implements to challenge the patient's proprioceptive system. The study found a greater number of successful results

Functional testing algorithm **Rehabilitation emphasis**

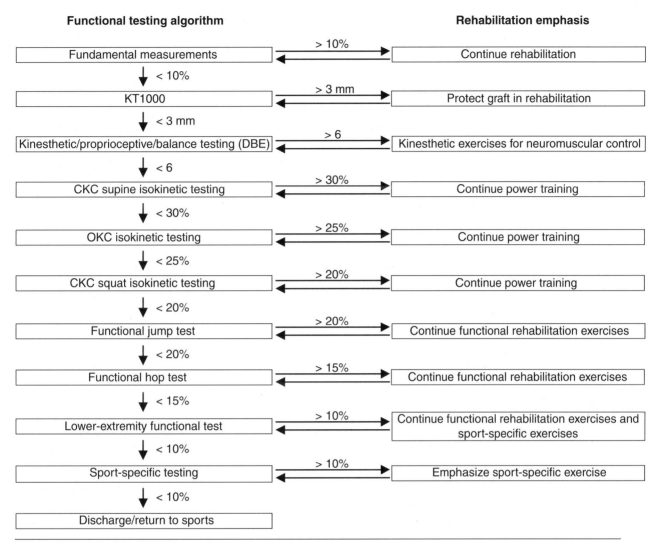

Figure 5.1 Functional testing algorithm as the foundation for a progressive rehabilitation program.

in the group that performed both traditional rehabilitation and perturbation training.

Open Kinetic Chain Isokinetic Testing

If the patient demonstrates deficits during open kinetic chain isokinetic testing, the focus should be on the individual components of the kinetic chain that have weaknesses (Gleim et al. 1978; Nicholas et al. 1976).

If weaknesses are present, rehabilitation focuses on open kinetic chain isolated muscle group training. This can be done using many exercise variations, including isometrics, isotonics, and isokinetics. Biofeedback training can probably help the patient with appropriate timing and muscle recruitment patterns. Closed kinetic chain total-extremity functional patterning exercises are also incorporated at this point to try to enhance the isolated muscle strength and to help the isolated muscle work in harmony with the functional movement.

Open kinetic chain isokinetic testing attends to weak individual segments in the kinetic chain.

Closed Kinetic Chain Squat Isokinetic Testing

The patient progresses to rehabilitation techniques that emphasize weight-bearing activities. Numerous exercises can be included at this time:

- Wall slides with two-leg eccentric lowering followed by two-leg concentric extension
- Wall slides with involved-leg eccentric lowering followed by two-leg concentric extension
- Wall slides with involved-leg eccentric lowering followed by involved-leg concentric extension
- Numerous squat variations (partial, lunge, etc.)
- Slide board
- Treadmill
- Elliptical runner

Emphasis is placed on single-leg closed kinetic chain exercises for the involved extremity based on the recent research by Neitzel et al. (2000), described earlier in this chapter. Open kinetic chain isolated-muscle rehabilitation exercises are also used at this time.

Functional Jump Testing

There is a major change in the focus of the patient's training or rehabilitation program when it progresses from controlled, proactive exercises to uncontrolled, reactive types of exercises. The emphasis in the training or rehabilitation program now includes two-leg activities, progressing from concentric movement patterns (where the patient initiates the movement) to eccentric deceleration movement patterns. During the eccentric deceleration movement, the patient must control the action reactively.

These are examples of exercises that are incorporated into the rehabilitation program at this point:

- Balance board
  1. Catching
  2. Throwing
- Slide board
  1. Catching
  2. Throwing
- Supine plyometrics on a leg-press system
  1. Straight
  2. Quadrant, clockwise
  3. Quadrant, counterclockwise
  4. Quadrant, random touches
- Basic plyometrics with the use of tape
  1. Anterior to posterior: fast feet, power
  2. Lateral ricochets: fast feet, power

  3. Anterior zigzags

  4. Sideway plyometrics

  5. Rotational activities

- Velocity-building, tubing-resisted plyometrics

  1. Anterior to posterior

  2. Lateral ricochets

  3. Diagonals

  4. Rotational activities

Hop Test

Since the hop test involves single-leg movements, many of the movements described under the jump test are now applied to the involved extremity alone.

Summary

Numerous functional activities involving the lower extremity require the use of closed kinetic chain movements. Several recent studies were described that provide the scientific basis for the application and efficacy of closed kinetic chain exercises. The next chapter describes the use of closed kinetic chain exercises in the rehabilitation of the upper extremity.

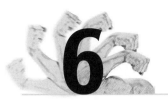

6

Closed Kinetic Chain Exercise for Rehabilitation and Conditioning of the Upper Extremity

Most of the activities of the upper extremity occur in what has traditionally been described as an open kinetic chain environment. Upper-extremity sport movement patterns, such as the tennis serve and throwing a baseball, occur with the distal segment of the upper extremity free to move and with the shoulder joint rotating at velocities ranging between 2,500°/s to well over 8,000°/s (Dillman 1991; Fleisig et al. 1995). Despite analyses of the upper extremity detailing a predominance of upper-extremity open chain function, clinicians have been using closed kinetic chain exercise to rehabilitate and strengthen the upper-extremity kinetic chain (Lephart and Henry 1996). Many sports, such as wrestling and gymnastics, and activities of daily living have significant closed kinetic chain components, where the hand is fixed and supporting body weight. These are integral components of normal human function. Therefore, it is important to consider the use of closed kinetic chain exercise and testing for the upper extremity in both rehabilitation and performance enhancement.

The important roles of the scapulothoracic and glenohumeral articulations and their interrelationship in upper-extremity movement justify the use of closed kinetic chain exercise. The vital interplay between these joints, termed the *scapulohumeral rhythm* (Inman et al. 1944), relies on coordinated dynamic muscular control of the scapula to ensure that scapular upward rotation occurs with

Scapular plane is the plane of the body 30° anterior to the frontal or coronal plane of the body.

changes in humeral elevation in the scapular plane (Codman 1934; Doody et al. 1970). Steindler (1955) observed that open kinetic chain exercises exhibit speed and emphasize free movement and less stabilization and that closed kinetic chain exercises involve greater stabilization and less acceleration. Closed kinetic chain exercises for the upper extremity involve the inherent stabilization of the scapulothoracic joint and co-contraction of the scapular stabilizers (Ellenbecker and Cappel 2000; Lephart and Henry 1996; Wilk, Arrigo et al. 1996).

Upper-Extremity Closed Kinetic Chain Exercise

Rehabilitation and conditioning exercises for the upper extremity and specifically the glenohumeral joint have traditionally focused on open kinetic chain movements. The literature provides several excellent EMG research studies that quantify the muscular activity levels inherent in these open kinetic chain exercises (Ballantyne et al. 1993; Blackburn et al. 1990; Hintermeister et al. 1998; Malanga et al. 1996; Townsend et al. 1991). These studies give the clinician specific guidelines for progression of exercise and an ability to isolate or emphasize a particular muscle group.

EMG Research

Significantly fewer EMG studies have been published on upper-extremity closed kinetic chain exercise than open kinetic chain exercises. Moseley et al. (1992) published a comprehensive analysis of the scapular muscles during traditional exercises used in rehabilitation programs. The exercises they studied included mainly open chain exercises but did include two closed chain exercises, the "push-up with a plus" and the press-up. The push-up with a plus involves the addition of maximal scapular protraction during the end of the ascent phase of the push-up. This plus position has been shown to result in high levels of muscular activity in the serratus anterior muscle. These exercises are detailed in chapter 8 on pages 91 and 95, respectively. Table 6.1 shows the EMG activity of the primary muscles used during these exercises, according to Moseley et al. (1992). The push-up with a plus demonstrated high activation levels of the middle and lower portions of the serratus anterior: 80% and 72% of maximal levels, respectively. The primary feature recommended in this exercise is the plus position, which produces maximal levels of scapular protraction and hence greater levels of serratus anterior activation than the traditional push-up position without a plus (Moseley et al. 1992). The other exercise featured in the article was the press-up, which produced high levels of activation of the pectoralis minor muscle but did not elicit high levels of muscular activity in the serratus anterior or trapezius musculature (Moseley et al. 1992). This study provides an excellent objective rationale for the use of these two closed kinetic chain upper-extremity exercises and information about the scapular muscles activated during their performance.

Decker et al. (1999) confirmed the importance of the plus position for serratus anterior activity. They measured the muscular activity patterns of the serratus anterior using EMG and found the push-up with a plus to elicit the highest levels of serratus activity among the seven open and closed kinetic chain rehabilitation exercises studied. These researchers concluded that exercises maintaining upward scapular rotation and accentuated scapular protraction produce the highest levels of serratus muscular activity.

Table 6.1	Muscular Activation Levels During the "Push-Up With a Plus" Closed Kinetic Chain Exercise	
Muscle group	**% MMT activity***	**Description**
Middle serratus anterior	80%	During plus maneuver
Lower serratus anterior	72%	Chest moving away from floor
Pectoralis minor	58%	During plus maneuver

* % MMT activity = percentage of muscular activity relative to maximal manual muscle test.

From Moseley et al. 1992.

Weiser et al. (1999) studied the effects of a simulated position of scapular protraction on glenohumeral joint stability and stress to the anterior glenohumeral joint capsular ligaments. Results showed a decrease in anterior humeral head translation in cadaveric specimens placed under a 15-N anteriorly directed load between conditions of neutral scapular positioning (6.3 mm of translation), 10° of protraction (4.1 mm of translation), and 20° of protraction (2.5 mm of translation). These findings indicate that increases in scapular protraction afford increased glenohumeral joint stability due to tension on the anterior ligamentous structures (O'Brien et al. 1990). Therefore, in addition to increased serratus anterior muscular activity (Decker et al. 1999; Moseley et al. 1992), greater inherent stability is also a characteristic of this position. This has clinical ramifications for applying closed kinetic chain upper-extremity exercises, particularly for individuals with glenohumeral joint instability.

Kibler et al. (1995) published EMG data from several closed kinetic chain exercises. The exercises studied included very low-intensity exercises such as weight-bearing weight shifts, rocker board exercises used early in both nonoperative and postoperative rehabilitation, and standard and angled push-ups. The muscular activity levels measured with EMG are listed in table 6.2 for the rotator cuff, deltoid, and scapular muscles. While activation levels are relatively low for many of the exercises, the primary inherent characteristic of muscular coactivation is demonstrated by this analysis. The rotator cuff and scapular stabilizers are activated but at lower levels than during many open kinetic chain exercises studied by Moseley et al. (1992). Of particular importance in many rehabilitation programs is the activation of the lower trapezius (Ballantyne et al. 1993; Blackburn et al. 1990; Townsend et al. 1991). The lower trapezius functions as an important scapular stabilizer by producing scapular depression, adduction, and upward rotation (Daniels and Worthingham 1986). Additionally, the lower trapezius has been identified as an important eccentric decelerator during the follow-through phase of the overhead throwing motion (DiGiovine et al. 1994). Closed chain exercises activate the lower trapezius and other scapular stabilizers. However, additional exercises that create higher levels of muscular activation of this important muscle are clearly warranted in rehabilitation and performance-enhancement programs.

Finally, Dillman et al. (1994) published an article introducing alternative classifications and nomenclature for rehabilitative exercise (see chapter 1 for details). They presented a case study that compared a push-up and wall push (FEL, or fixed external load, exercises), which traditionally are classified as closed

Table 6.2 Muscle Firing as a Percentage of Maximal Muscular Activity for Different Closed Chain Patterns

Activity	Serratus anterior	Supra-spinatus	Infra-spinatus	Rhomboid	Upper trapezius	Lower trapezius	Anterior deltoid	Posterior deltoid
Standing weight shift	< 10	< 10	< 10	< 10	< 10	< 10	< 10	< 10
Standing rocking board	< 10	< 10	< 10	< 10	< 10	< 10	< 10	< 10
Four-point weight shift	30	< 10	< 10	< 10	< 10	< 10	30	< 10
Four-point rocking board	30	< 10	< 10	< 10	< 10	< 10	30	< 10
Clock flexion	20	20	20	20	20	< 10	20	< 10
Clock abduction	20	20	20	40	20	< 10	20	< 10
Standard push-up	25	20	20	35	35	10	70	30
Angled push-up	25	20	20	35	35	10	45	30

From Kibler et al. 1995.

kinetic chain exercises, with a bench press and arm press at different loads (MEL, or moving external load, exercises). The results of their case study show that these exercises have similar biomechanical characteristics and similar EMG activity patterns in the rotator cuff, deltoids, and pectoralis musculature. Because this was a case study, no definitive statements regarding average muscular activity patterns can be gleaned from this study.

A follow-up study by Blackard et al. (1999) compared the standard push-up (FEL) with the bench press with comparable body-weight loading (MEL) and with the bench press with no load (MNL, movable boundary with no external load). This study showed no significant difference in EMG activity of the pectoralis major and triceps musculature during the equally loaded exercises, despite different boundary (open vs. closed chain) conditions. These results agree with the earlier case study of Dillman et al. (1994), which found that the biomechanical characteristics of upper-extremity exercise are strikingly similar between boundary conditions when comparable loads are applied. Therefore, these studies show very similar muscular activity patterns in the open and closed chain upper-extremity movement patterns studied. Clearly, further study of the effects of upper-extremity closed kinetic chain exercises on more muscles and on the activity of musculature in adjoining segments (i.e., crossing the scapulothoracic articulation) is needed before a greater, more definitive conclusion can be reached.

Anatomical Considerations

One of the primary considerations in the application of upper-extremity closed kinetic chain exercise is the anatomy of the scapulothoracic, glenohumeral, ulnohumeral, radiohumeral, and intercarpal joints. The anatomical features of the scapulothoracic joint applicable in closed kinetic chain exercise pertain primarily to static posture and dynamic stabilization. The static posture of the human scapulothoracic joint is often altered in unilaterally dominant athletes (Ellenbecker and Derscheid 1989; Kulund et al. 1979; Priest and Nagel 1976). The dominant shoulder and scapulothoracic joint are significantly lower than the nondominant shoulder and scapulothoracic joint (Kulund et al. 1979; Priest and Nagel 1976). While the exact mechanism that causes this lower dominant shoulder (termed *tennis shoulder)* is not completely understood, it involves increased scapular protraction, downward rotation, and depression. Additionally, the inferior and medial borders of the scapula often protrude posteriorly off the thoracic wall, a condition termed *scapular winging* (Kibler 1998a; Zeier 1973). Scapular winging has been attributed to weakness of the serratus anterior and lower trapezius musculature (Kibler 1998a) and to pathology of the nerve innervating the serratus anterior, the long thoracic nerve (Kibler 1998a; Zeier 1973). Normally, the bilateral difference in the distance between the inferior angle of the scapula and the corresponding vertebral spinous process in the transverse plane is within 1 to 1.5 cm. This measurement, termed the *lateral scapular slide* by Kibler (1991, 1998a, 1998b), has been used as a clinical measure to detect deficient dynamic scapular control or stabilization (Litchfield et al. 1998). Identification of a bilateral difference of more than 1 to 1.5 cm indicates the inclusion of exercises to address deficiencies in dynamic muscular scapular stabilization. Due to the increase in proximal upper-extremity loading inherent in closed kinetic chain exercise, the postural and positional relationships of the scapula become important variables for evaluation.

Perhaps the most important anatomical relationships to consider for closed kinetic chain exercise for the upper extremity are in the glenohumeral joint. The exact orientation of the glenoid fossa, especially with respect to the humeral head, is of critical importance when using closed kinetic chain exercises in individuals with glenohumeral joint instability, rotator cuff dysfunction, and osteoarthritic degenerative conditions. The recommendation for applying closed kinetic chain exercise to shoulder pathologies is to minimize shear force and humeral head translation and to increase true compressive forces in the glenohumeral joint. To accomplish this, the clinician must understand the anatomical orientation of the joint surfaces.

The human glenoid fossa is oriented slightly inferiorly with the arms held at the sides (Poppen and Walker 1976) and tilted anteriorly 30° from the true coronal plane of the body (Saha 1983). This anterior version of the glenoid fossa coupled with the 30° of retrotorsion of the humeral head aligns the glenohumeral joint's articulating surfaces optimally, with maximal bony congruity when the arm is positioned 30° anteriorly to the coronal plane (Saha 1983). This positioning, termed the *scapular plane,* is commonly used and universally recommended as a position of exercise based on the principles of osseous congruity, ligamentous stability, musculotendinous length–tension relationships, and functional ramifications (Saha 1983). Understanding these important anatomical relationships, the clinician should use closed kinetic chain exercise positions where the shoulder is placed in the scapular plane and aligned to minimize shear and translatory forces.

Recent research has demonstrated the important role that glenohumeral joint compression plays in decreasing shear and humeral head translation. Warner et al. (1999) studied the effects of applying 5, 25, and 50 pounds (22, 111, and 222 N) of compressive force to cadaveric glenohumeral joints. The joint compression resulted in decreases in joint translation at neutral elevation from 11 mm to 2 mm between 5 and 25 pounds (22 and 111 N) of compression. At 45° of abduction in the scapular plane, humeral head translation was reduced from 21.5 mm to 1.4 mm between 5 and 25 pounds (22 and 111 N) of joint compression. The results of this study demonstrate the positive effects of glenohumeral joint compression in controlling humeral head translation and have significant clinical ramifications,

Lateral scapular slide test, developed by Ben Kibler, MD, measures the static position of the human scapula, using the distance from the vertebral spinous process to the inferior angle of the scapula.

particularly when working with individuals with glenohumeral joint instability or shoulder injuries. An increase in true glenohumeral joint surface compression can be accomplished and is encouraged in many rehabilitative exercise applications.

The pathological effects of superior migration of the humeral head within the glenoid have been well documented (Chen et al. 1999; Neer 1983). Performance of closed kinetic chain exercises with the arm in lower, less functional positions of abduction (arms close to the side or adducted) can create superior migration in the absence of optimal dynamic humeral head control or stabilization or asymmetric capsular flexibility (Harryman et al. 1990). The exercises in chapter 8 apply these important concepts, using functional positions of elevation in the scapular plane to create an optimal closed kinetic chain environment during exercise.

Donkers et al. (1993) studied the forces acting on the elbow during a push-up exercise. The peak compressive force at the ulnohumeral joint is equal to 45% of body weight with the hands placed in the normal push-up position. These researchers reported that the elbow compressive forces were decreased when the hands were placed either further apart or in a more superior position. A one-arm push-up increased compressive force by 31% when compared with a two-arm push-up. Valgus torque increased by 54% with the hands in a superior position and by 42% when a one-arm push-up was performed. The greatest force on the elbow results when the elbow is flexed approximately 30° (Werner and An 1994). This force approaches three times body weight. This biomechanical information allows clinicians to better understand the type of loads and stresses placed across the human elbow joint during closed kinetic chain loading.

Morrey and An (1983) experimentally demonstrated the superior osseous and ligamentous stability of the ulnohumeral joint. Placement of the elbow in an extended position during most closed kinetic chain exercises for the upper extremity ensures collective stability from both the osseous congruity and ligamentous structures. The elbow at or near complete extension requires less stability from the ligaments and dynamic structures and maximizes the contribution from the bony ulnohumeral configuration (Morrey and An 1983).

Pressure through the intercarpal (wrist) joints during closed kinetic chain exercise is acknowledged; however, no formal investigation clearly measuring muscular function or joint loads is presently available. Careful placement of the wrist and hand and limitation of extended periods of training with the wrist held in end-range extension in the closed kinetic chain environment are clinically recommended. Alteration of wrist position through the use of rehabilitative devices, explained in chapter 8, can help individuals perform upper-extremity closed kinetic chain exercise while minimizing the stress to the wrist.

Upper-Extremity Closed Kinetic Chain Training

Research that reports the effects of closed chain upper-extremity training is sparse, despite its current widespread use in rehabilitation and exercise training. However, two studies have examined the effects of the addition of upper-extremity closed kinetic chain training to traditional open kinetic chain rehabilitation programs (Lephart et al. 1998; McGee et al. 1999). Lephart et al. (1998) used five neuromuscular control exercises that emphasized joint positioning, joint approximation and compression, and muscular coactivation in one experimental group in addition to traditional open kinetic chain shoulder exercises in subjects with anterior glenohumeral joint instability. They found significant improvements in kinesthetic ability, lateral scapular slide testing at 120° of abduction, and isokinetically documented protraction and retraction strength in the experimental group following the addition of closed kinetic chain exercise. No significant improvements were documented in these parameters in the training group that performed only open kinetic chain upper-extremity exercise or in the control group. These results clearly support the use of upper-extremity closed kinetic chain exercise in individuals with anterior glenohumeral joint instability.

McGee et al. (1999) performed a prospective, randomized, controlled clinical trial comparing the effects of traditional open kinetic chain rehabilitation exercises and traditional exercises plus a closed kinetic chain exercise program using a balance board in a group of patients diagnosed with shoulder impingement. These researchers found significant decreases in subjective pain ratings, improved functional status using rating scales, and improved isokinetic strength scores for the internal and external rotators. However, no significant difference was measured between groups. A major limitation of this study was the small sample size in each group, which probably limited the ability to demonstrate statistical significance. While closed kinetic chain training in this study did produce subjective, objective, and functional improvements, these improvements did not differ from subjects diagnosed with glenohumeral joint impingement who performed only traditional open kinetic chain training. Further research is clearly needed to better understand the effects of closed kinetic chain training in patients with different upper-extremity problems.

Upper-Extremity Closed Kinetic Chain Testing

There is also a paucity of research on upper-extremity closed kinetic chain testing. The physical education and rehabilitative literature shows that the primary true closed kinetic chain test used for the upper extremity has been the push-up. Roetert et al. (1992) used the number of push-ups performed in 30 seconds and 1 minute by elite junior tennis players as a measure of upper-extremity strength and endurance. Specific characteristics of the push-up were the consistent descent to a position of elbow flexion in which the upper arm was grossly parallel to the testing surface (Roetert et al. 1992; Roetert and Ellenbecker 1998). Descriptive data has been presented for the push-up test for elite junior tennis players but has limited use outside of physical training and rehabilitation of that specific population (Roetert and Ellenbecker 1998).

Davies and Dickhoff-Hoffman (1993) described a modification of the standard push-up that they termed the closed kinetic chain upper-extremity stability test. An individual begins the test in a standard push-up position, with the hands on two parallel pieces of tape 3 feet (0.9 m) apart, below the shoulders. The individual is instructed to move both hands as rapidly as possible from one tape line to the other, touching each line alternately in a "windshield wiper" fashion (figure 6.1). The number of line touches in 15 seconds is recorded using a stopwatch for objective quantification of upper-extremity closed kinetic chain function. Goldbeck and Davies (2000) recently completed a test-retest reliability study of this closed chain upper-extremity stability test. Subjects were tested twice using identical methodology, resulting in a reliability coefficient of .927, indicating that this test is a highly reliable clinical evaluation tool. The average number of line touches for the 24 male college students in the study was 27.8 ± 1.77 for the pretest and 27.9 ± 1.97 for the retest.

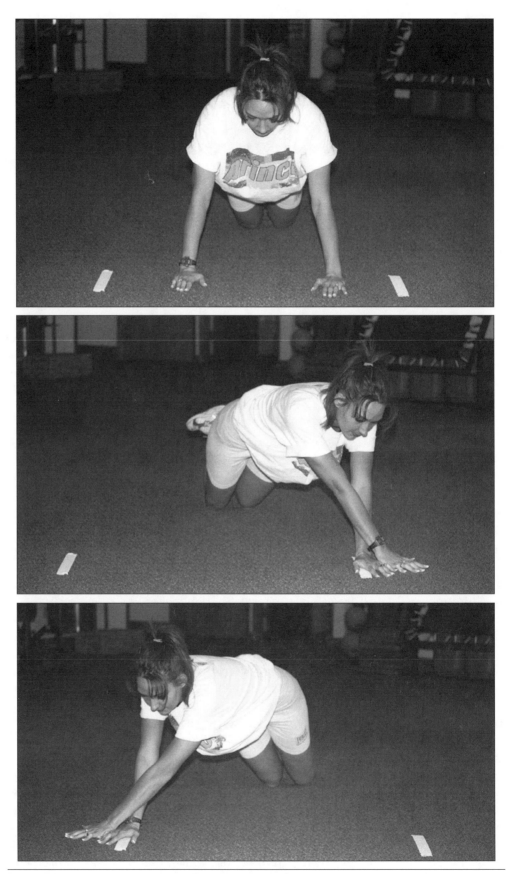

Figure 6.1 Closed kinetic chain upper-extremity stability test.

Closed Kinetic Chain Upper-Extremity Stability Test

Patient name: _____ GC#: _____ Date of birth: _____

MD: _____ PT: _____ D.O.S./D.O.I.: _____

Diagnosis: _____ Height: _____ in. Weight: _____ lb

Procedure

1. Subject assumes push-up (male) or modified push-up on knees (female) position.
2. Subject moves both hands back and forth from each line as many times as possible in 15 seconds. Lines are 3 feet (0.9 m) apart.
3. Count the number of lines touched by both hands.
4. Begin with one submaximal warm-up. Repeat three times and average.
5. Normalize score by applying the following formula:

   Score = $\dfrac{\text{Average number of lines touched}}{\text{Height (in.)}}$

6. Determine power by applying the following formula (68% = trunk, head, arms):

   Power = $\dfrac{68\% \text{ body weight} \times \text{average number of lines touched}}{15 \text{ s}}$

Data

Date _____

	1	2	3	Average
Touches				

Score_____

Power_____

Date _____

	1	2	3	Average
Touches				

Score_____

Power_____

Date _____

	1	2	3	Average
Touches				

Score_____

Power_____

Date _____

	1	2	3	Average
Touches				

Score_____

Power_____

Norm	Male (average)	Female (average)
Touches	14.5	20.5
Power	150	135
Score	.26	.31

The CKC UE Stability Test form contains the specific instructions for administering the closed kinetic chain upper-extremity stability test, as well as normative data for both males and females. Data is normalized on this test for males and females by dividing the number of line touches by the subject's height in inches. The reason for normalizing the number of touches to the patient's height is the fixed distance of the targets that need to be touched. The test could also be performed so it would be consistent for all patients by placing the two lines a distance apart equal to a specified percentage of the patient's height. This would require changing the distance between the two lines each time the test is performed, which would be inefficient in a busy clinical setting. Therefore, instead of changing the target distances for each person, the distance is kept constant, and the performance data is normalized by the patient's height. This normalization also eliminates the biomechanical advantage that a taller person has and allows accurate comparison of the performance data among subjects.

Power scores can also be calculated for the closed kinetic chain upper-extremity stability test. Subjects of different body weights produce different amounts of power. For example, a person who weighs 100 pounds and touches 23 times has different power capabilities than a subject who weighs 200 pounds and touches 23 times. Multiplying 68% of the subject's body weight (the superincumbent weight of the upper extremities, head, and trunk) in pounds by the number of touches and dividing by 15 seconds gives the power.

$$\text{Power} = \frac{68\% \text{ body weight (lb)} \times \text{touches}}{15 \text{ s}}$$

The values are divided by 15 seconds because that is the time of the test. To calculate a power score, the total work performed must be divided by the time it took to perform the work.

A time-based platform is a device that calculates the force applied in various directions and the amount of time that force is exhibited.

Additional upper-extremity closed kinetic chain testing research was reported by Ellenbecker and Roetert (1996) and Ellenbecker and Mattalino (1997). A Fastex device, a circular time-based platform with pressure-sensitive piezoelectric film around the perimeter, was used to quantify closed chain stance stability. This closed chain stance stability test consisted of a 20-second bout of a unilateral upper-extremity stance (figure 6.2). The contralateral arm was positioned in the lumbar spine region to minimize compensation by that extremity. The feet were positioned 1 foot (0.3 m) apart. An 80° arm–trunk angle was standardized using a universal goniometer. A bilateral comparison was made of the amount of postural sway or perturbation measured by the device, and a total average stability parameter was generated to represent the ability of the subject to remain still or stable while balancing on the stationary platform. Subjects closed their eyes during testing to minimize the effects or bias from visual stimulus and feedback. Subjects were told to remain "as still as possible" during the 20-second testing period. A larger score represented an increase in the amount of sway or imbalance during the testing period.

Using this closed chain stance stability test, Ellenbecker and Roetert (1996) tested 19 professional baseball pitchers and 75 elite junior tennis players. The bilateral comparison of unilateral stance stability showed no significant difference between extremities in this closed chain test. This finding is in contrast to previous open kinetic chain testing in these unilaterally dominant athletes. Dominant-arm shoulder internal rotation, extension, adduction, elbow extension, wrist flexion and extension, and forearm pronation were consistently documented as stronger relative to the nondominant extremity with isolated

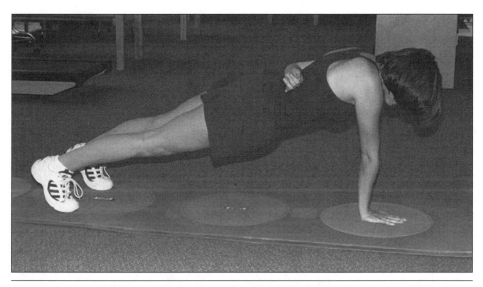

Figure 6.2 Unilateral closed chain stance stability test using Fastex.

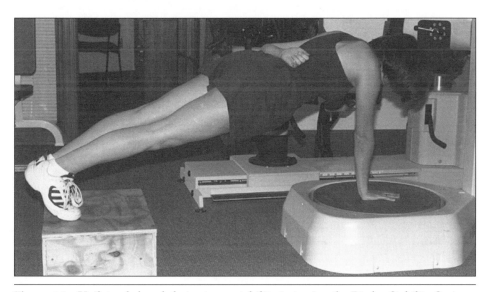

Figure 6.3 Unilateral closed chain stance stability test using the Biodex Stability System.

isokinetic testing in elite junior tennis players and professional baseball pitchers (Ellenbecker 1991, 1992; Ellenbecker et al. 1999; Wilk et al. 1993).

Additional research compared open kinetic chain isokinetic shoulder internal and external rotation testing in the modified base position with unilateral closed chain stance stability in patients with glenohumeral joint instability and impingement (Ellenbecker and Mattalino 1997). This study found no significant correlation between the bilateral comparisons using closed chain testing and open kinetic chain internal and external rotation testing. The presence of a significant deficit in open kinetic chain internal or external rotation strength did not statistically correlate with a deficit in unilaterally assessed closed kinetic chain stance stability. This research indicates that closed kinetic chain testing may provide additional unique information that is distinct from that provided by open kinetic chain testing in the upper extremity and that closed kinetic chain testing has an important part in a complete rehabilitation or performance training program.

One of the authors of this book (Ellenbecker) is replicating the studies of Ellenbecker and Roetert (1996) and Ellenbecker and Mattalino (1997) using alternative technologies. An example, displayed in figure 6.3, is the Biodex Stability System, which provides an objective way to assess lower- and upper-extremity closed chain stance stability.

Summary

Despite the paucity of research on closed chain upper-extremity exercises, the anatomical and biomechanical factors discussed in this chapter clearly indicate the potential benefits and effectiveness of closed chain upper-extremity exercise and testing. Further research must be performed to better understand the exact muscular activation patterning, benefits of training, and optimal methods to monitor and measure functional performance in the closed chain environment. The information presented in this chapter underlies the application of the upper-extremity closed kinetic chain exercises presented in chapter 8.

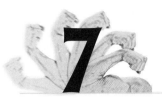

7

Lower-Extremity Closed Kinetic Chain Exercises

This chapter presents several closed kinetic chain exercises for the lower extremity that are recommended for both rehabilitation and performance-enhancement training. A thorough evaluation must be performed to determine whether these exercises are appropriate for the individual. The order and progression of the exercises will vary according to individual needs and deficiencies. Careful monitoring of an individual's signs and symptoms is important in determining progression of these exercises.

Each exercise for the lower extremity will be presented with exercise name, start position, exercise action, purpose, primary muscles used, indications, contraindications, and pearls of performance listed where indicated.

Linea Closed Kinetic Chain Isokinetic Exercise

Start position: With the lower extremities in either a flexed or extended position

Exercise action: Use a bilateral lower-extremity reciprocal isokinetic pattern.

Purpose: To capitalize on isokinetic resistance, which involves a movement at a fixed velocity with an accommodating resistance. This allows strengthening the entire lower-extremity kinetic chain in a partially or fully weight-bearing position.

Primary muscles used: Gluteus maximus, hamstrings, quadriceps, gastrocnemius

Indications: Allows early submaximal exercises following an injury or surgery. The accommodating resistance, used in an appropriate manner, prevents overloading the muscle or joint. This exercise and position is also useful for a patient who is bearing only partial weight due to an injury or a postsurgical condition.

Contraindications: If joint motion should not be permitted or if exercises should be performed in an open kinetic chain pattern

Pearls of performance: The Linea computerized isokinetic dynamometer is particularly useful in a clinical setting where objective performance testing needs to be performed regularly to assess the status of a patient following an injury. Performance on these tests often provides guidance for the rehabilitation program.

The Linea can also be used in a variety of muscle training modes. The Linea allows isometric, isotonic, and isokinetic resistance patterns and can also be set to use isometric, concentric, or eccentric muscle actions.

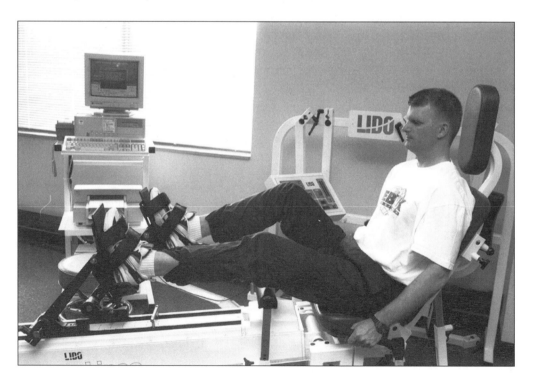

Versa Climber

Start position: Sitting, using the arms, or standing, using the arms and legs

Exercise action: Use either the upper extremities in a sitting position or the upper and lower extremities simultaneously in a reciprocal, rhythmic pattern.

Purpose: To provide a general upper- and lower-body closed kinetic chain workout

Primary muscles used: Gluteus maximus, hamstrings, quadriceps, gastrocnemius, shoulder complex flexors and extensors; core stabilization

Indications: Can be used for just upper-extremity or a combination of upper- and lower-extremity muscular endurance training and cardiovascular training.

Contraindications: If joint movement is not permitted; if the patient should not bear weight; not for a deconditioned patient

Pearls of performance: Great total-body conditioning device

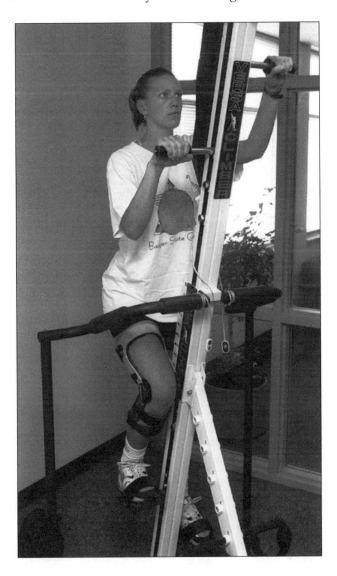

Frontal Plane Lateral Exercises

Start position: Standing on a balance or slide board

Exercise action: Move from side to side in the frontal plane using the leg abductors and adductors.

Purpose: To exercise muscles in the frontal plane and develop neuromuscular control in that direction; to strengthen the lower-extremity musculature

Primary muscles used: Hip abductors, hip adductors, hamstrings, quadriceps, and gluteus maximus

Indications: For anyone who performs activities that involve multiplane movement patterns

Contraindications: If joint movement is not permitted; if the patient should not bear weight; not for deconditioned patient, those with unstable joints in the frontal plane (e.g., knee medial collateral ligament (MCL) or lateral collateral ligament (LCL) injuries, patellofemoral subluxators), or patients with lateral overuse syndromes (i.e., iliotibial band (ITB) syndromes)

Pearls of performance: Good exercise for skiers because it replicates the skiing motion

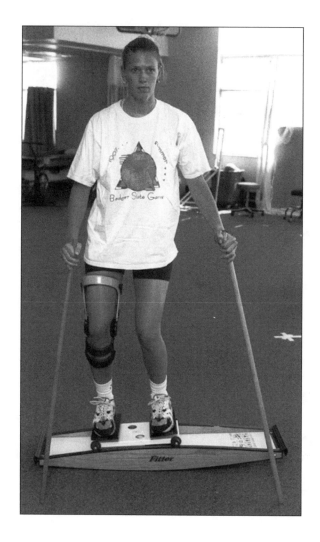

Squats and Plyometric Jumps

Squat Rack

Start position: Standing

Exercise action: Perform a squat.

Purpose: To develop the power of the lower-extremity musculature in a functional, weight-bearing position

Primary muscles used: Gluteus maximus, hamstrings, quadriceps, gastrocnemius

Indications: To improve strength in lower-extremity musculature

Contraindications: If joint motion should not be permitted or if exercises should be performed in an open kinetic chain pattern

Pearls of performance: Squats can be performed through different ranges of motion (e.g., 30°, 60°, 90°) depending on the individual's limitations.

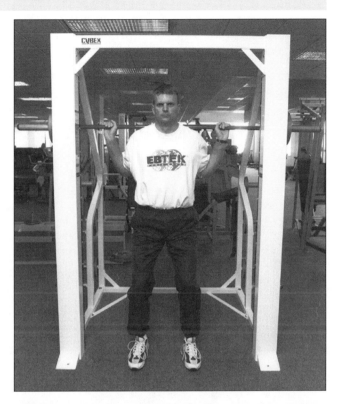

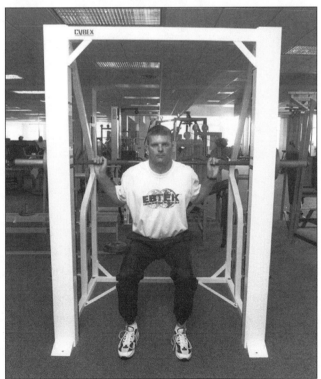

Plyometric Jump Boxes

Start position: Standing

Exercise action: Use plyometric stretch (i.e., eccentric prestretch followed by a concentric shortening action of the muscle).

Purpose: To capitalize on the benefits of plyometrics, which include facilitating the stretch to the muscle spindle and prestretching the series elastic components in the muscle to store kinetic energy to enhance the concentric muscle action, and to enhance performance

Primary muscles used: Gluteus maximus, hamstrings, quadriceps, gastrocnemius

Indications: Higher-performance training activity

Contraindications: If joint motion should not be permitted; if exercises should be performed in an open kinetic chain pattern; not for deconditioned patients or those with quadriceps weakness

Pearls of performance: One of the best training modes to enhance lower-extremity functional performance. Plyometrics is very versatile because of the many different forms and variations that can be used.

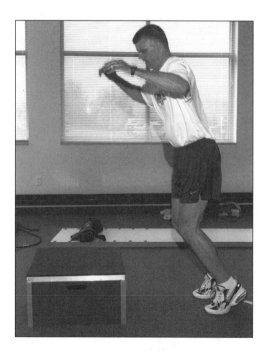

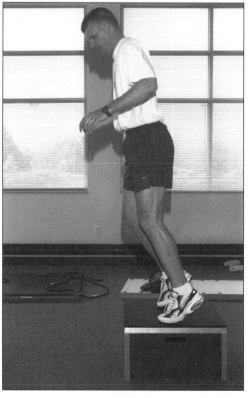

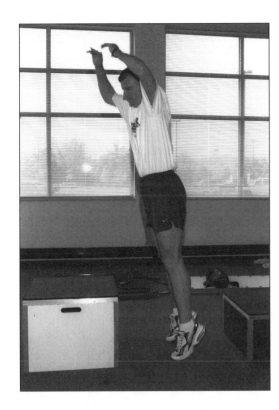

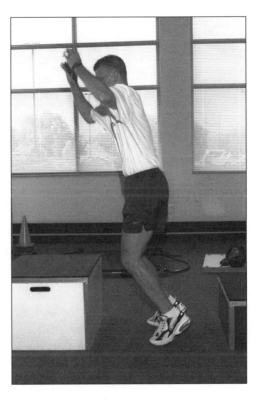

Velocity Builder

Start position: Standing with the chest harness on and the surgical tubing hooked to the harness

Exercise action: Can use squat movement patterns or plyometric exercises with several variations.

Purpose: To capitalize on the benefits of plyometrics, which include facilitating the stretch to the muscle spindle and prestretching the series elastic components in the muscle to store kinetic energy to enhance the concentric muscle action, and to enhance performance

Primary muscles used: Gluteus maximus, hamstrings, quadriceps, gastrocnemius

Indications: To strengthen the lower-extremity musculature, to develop power through the performance of plyometric movement patterns

Contraindications: Various lower-extremity pathologies, especially chondral injuries or effusion in the joints

Pearls of performance: The versatility allows one to use squat exercises and to progress to numerous variations of plyometric exercises.

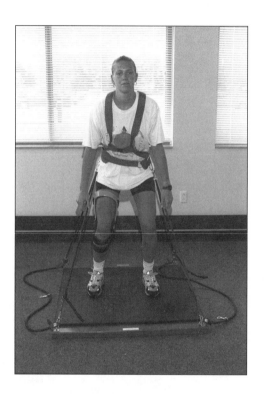 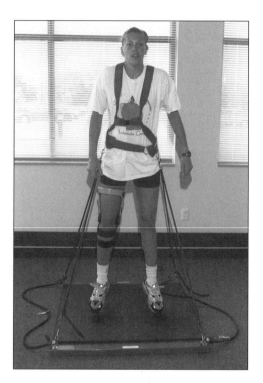

Tubing-Resisted Exercises

Start position: Standing with surgical tubing hooked to a belt or to a worn harness

Exercise action: Can perform various motions, such as resisted walking, power walking, or running, as well as many variations, such as side shuffles, cariocas, and so on.

Purpose: Specificity training to develop functional power by having the individual replicate functional activities

Primary muscles used: Gluteus maximus, hamstrings, quadriceps, gastrocnemius

Indications: Fun, functional specificity training

Contraindications: Significant dynamic activity to lower extremities

Pearls of performance: Can use many variations, from resisted stepping in place to running cariocas.

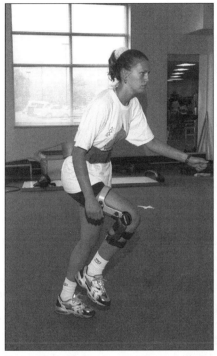 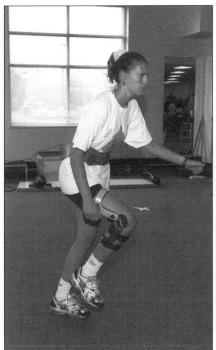 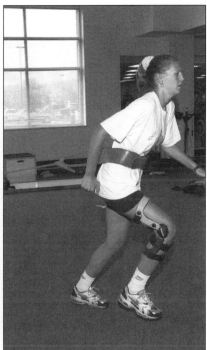

Forward running.

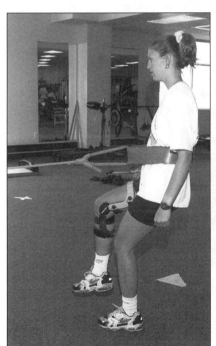 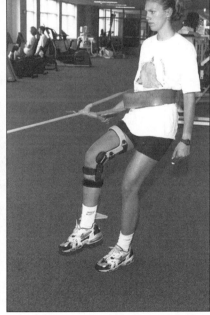

Retro running.

Wall Slides

Start position: Standing

Exercise action: Slide the back, which is supported to help provide stability, down the wall.

Purpose: Supported lower-extremity strengthening

Primary muscles used: Gluteus maximus, hamstrings, quadriceps, gastrocnemius

Indications: For early therapeutic intervention following an injury or surgery

Contraindications: Significant dynamic activity to lower extremities

Pearls of performance: Applies the principles of overload and progression. These are stages that can be used in the application of wall slides:

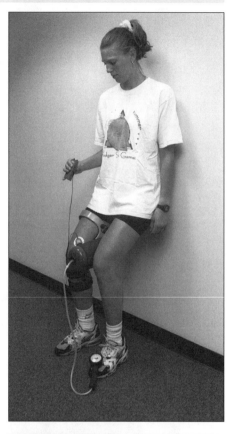

- From the upright, standing position, the individual performs two-leg eccentric lowering through the indicated range of motion, followed by a two-leg concentric contraction back to the upright starting position.
- The individual performs one-leg eccentric lowering through the indicated range of motion, followed by a two-leg concentric contraction.
- The individual performs one-leg eccentric lowering through the indicated range of motion, followed by a one-leg concentric contraction.

When the individual reaches the end of the range of motion for the flexion phase, the patellae should end up directly over the end of the toes.

Other common variations of this exercise include the use of biofeedback to attempt to selectively recruit certain muscles, such as the vastus medialis obliquus. A combination exercise in which the individual performs first an adductor squeeze and then a wall slide also attempts to selectively recruit the vastus medialis obliquus.

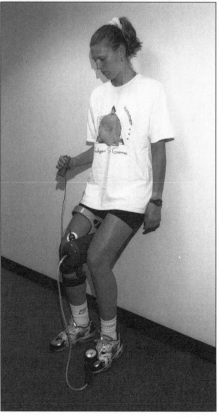

Agility Exercises

Agility Drills

Start position: Standing

Exercise action: Depends on specific desired performance

Purpose: To enhance specific functional performance

Primary muscles used: All lower-extremity muscles

Indications: To develop functional power

Contraindications: Significant dynamic activity to lower extremities

Pearls of performance: Unlimited exercises can be used, depending on the specific performance goals.

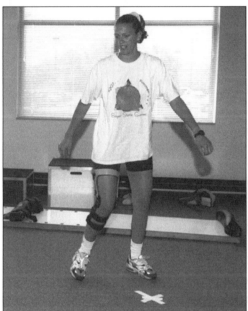
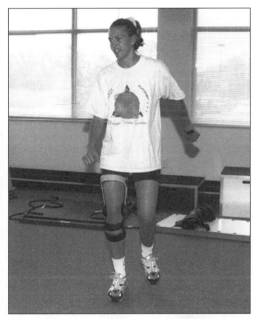
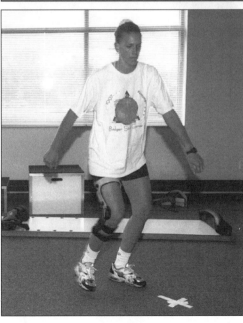
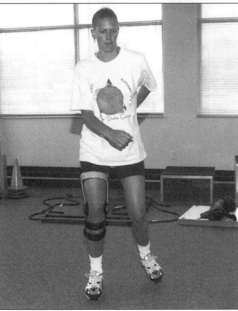

Fastex Interactive Computerized Functional Training

Start position: Standing

Exercise action: Numerous lower-extremity patterns can be performed.

Purpose: The computerization allows objective documentation of functional performance training and testing.

Primary muscles used: Hip ab/adductors, hip internal/external rotators, gluteus maximus, hamstrings, quadriceps, gastrocnemius

Indications: Objective documentation of functional lower-extremity patterns of many variations

Contraindications: Significant dynamic activity to lower extremities

Pearls of performance: Because of the versatility of the computer and Fastex setup, many variations of objective testing can be performed, from static standing balance to agility tests requiring multiple lower-extremity movement patterns. Fastex testing and training can be used to measure performance in replicated sport activities.

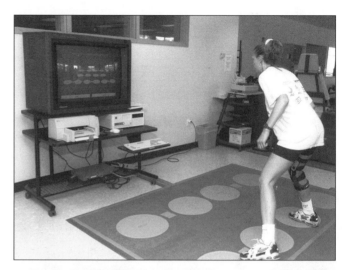

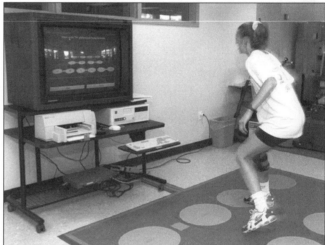

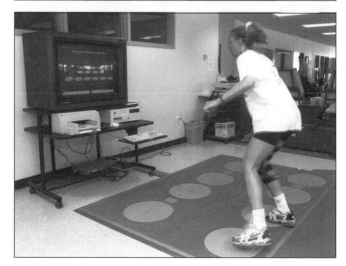

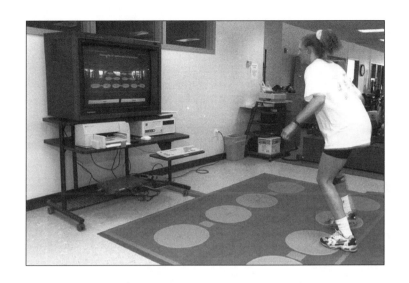

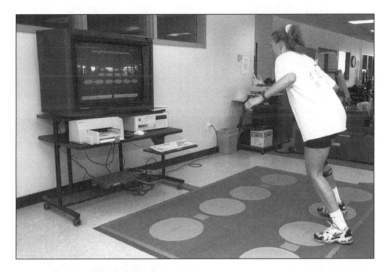

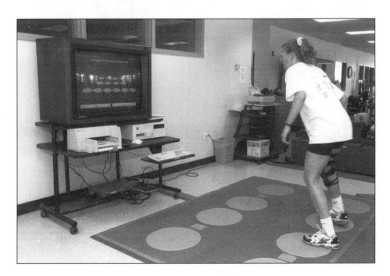

Squat Lunge Variations

Start position: Standing

Exercise action: Lunge in various directions, such as front, side, and diagonal lunges.

Purpose: To strengthen the lower-extremity muscles in different positions along the length–tension curve

Primary muscles used: Gluteus maximus, hamstrings, quadriceps, gastrocnemius

Contraindications: Significant dynamic activity to lower extremities

Pearls of performance: This exercise can be performed with just the body weight or with dumbbells in the hands to provide additional resistance for the overload training response.

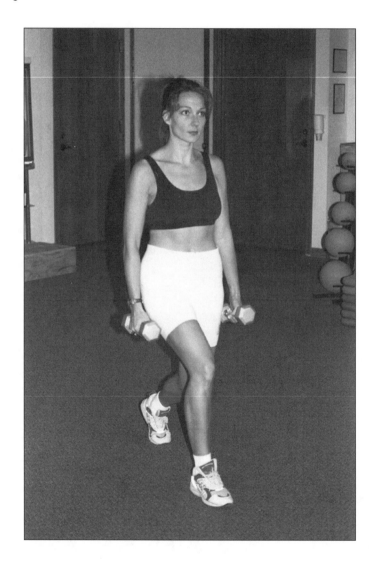

Balance Training

Single-Direction Balance Boards

Start position: Standing

Exercise action: Either maintain balance in a static position, or perform specific dynamic-balance exercises.

Purpose: To enhance lower-extremity proprioception/kinesthesia

Primary muscles used: Hip ab/adductors, hip internal/external rotators, gluteus maximus, hamstrings, quadriceps, gastrocnemius

Indications: Patients with joint injuries

Contraindications: Significant dynamic activity to lower extremities

Pearls of performance: Unlimited variations can be implemented using the principles of progression and overload. Here are examples of parameters that can be manipulated:

1. No weight bearing to partial to full weight bearing
2. Static-balance to dynamic-balance movement patterns
3. Single-plane movement patterns to multiplane movement patterns
5. Easy to more difficult and unstable boards
6. Double-leg to single-leg activities

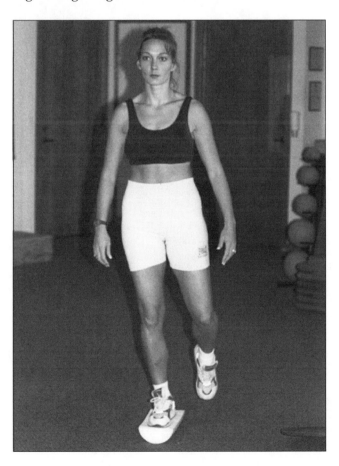

Multi-Direction Balance Boards

Start position: Standing

Exercise action: Either maintain balance in a static position, or perform specific dynamic-balance exercises.

Purpose: To enhance lower-extremity proprioception/kinesthesia

Primary muscles used: Hip ab/adduction, hip internal/external rotators, gluteus maximus, hamstrings, quadriceps, gastrocnemius

Indications: Patients with joint injuries

Contraindications: Significant dynamic activity to lower extremities

Pearls of performance: Same as for "Single-Direction Balance Boards"

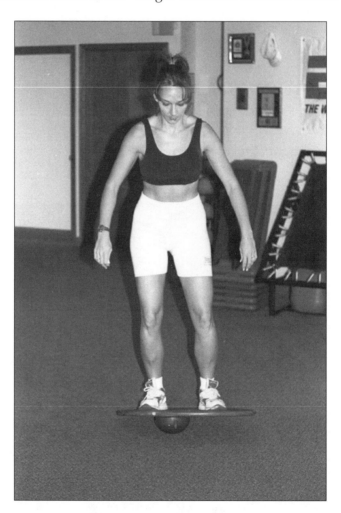

Leg Press

Start position: Supine

Exercise action: Tandem lower-extremity flexion-to-extension motions

Purpose: To strengthen the lower-extremity muscles when only partial weight bearing is permitted, analogous to submaximal training

Primary muscles used: Gluteus maximus, hamstrings, quadriceps, gastrocnemius

Indications: When only partial weight bearing is indicated, and to progress to heavier weights. It is also one of the best movement patterns to begin low-level plyometric exercises.

Contraindications: Significant dynamic activity to lower extremities

Pearls of performance: A pattern similar to that for the wall slide can be used. The individual can begin with a two-leg concentric contraction followed by a two-leg eccentric contraction. Progression is to a two-leg concentric contraction followed by a one-leg eccentric action. Finally, a single-leg concentric contraction followed by a single-leg eccentric action completes the progression.

Additionally, double- and single-leg plyometric exercises can be performed. A progression from straight plyometrics (touch and go) to quadrant plyometrics in clockwise and counterclockwise directions should be used. Quadrant plyometrics can also be performed in a random manner.

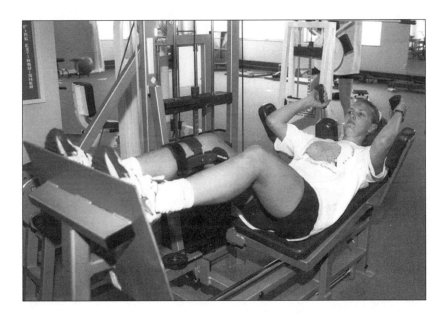

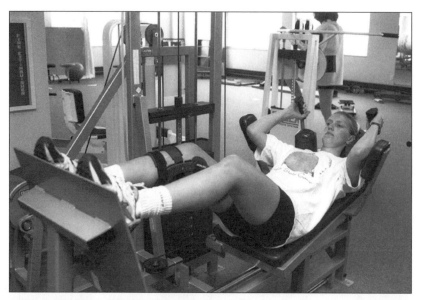

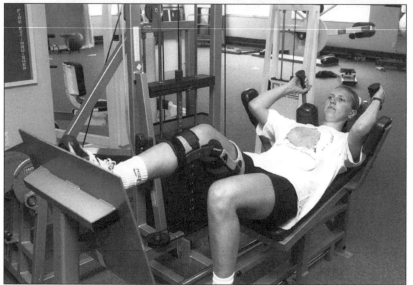

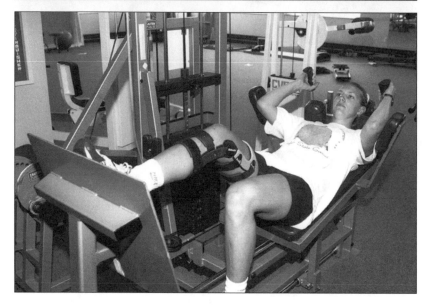

Elastic Resistance Exercises

Forward Step-Up and Step-Down

Start position: Standing in front of steps

Exercise action: Step straight ahead with the involved extremity.

Purpose: To strengthen muscles, to work on balance and coordination

Primary muscles used: Hip flexors, quadriceps, hip extensors

Indications: Individuals with lower-extremity weakness or with balance deficits

Contraindications: Significant dynamic activity to lower extremities

Pearls of performance: The individual can exercise the muscles concentrically during the step-up phase of the movement and then eccentrically during the lowering phase.

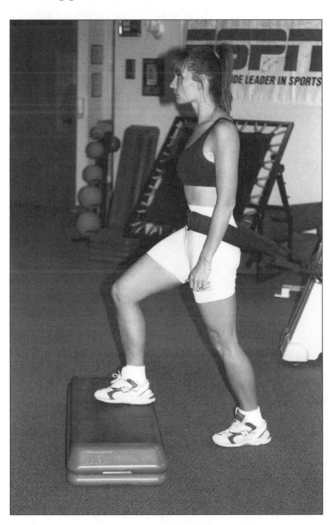

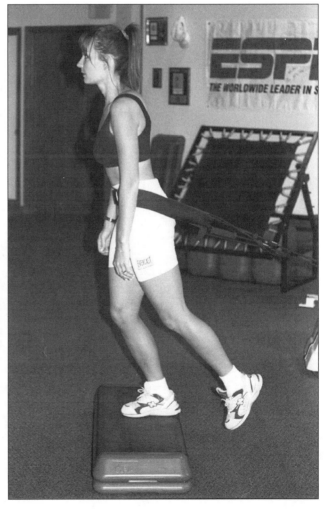

Retro Step-Up

Start position: Standing with back to the steps

Exercise action: Step up backward with the involved extremity.

Purpose: To strengthen lower-extremity muscles and to improve balance

Primary muscles used: Hip extensors, hamstrings, quadriceps

Indications: To strengthen posterior muscles, patients with anterior cruciate ligament (ACL) reconstructions, patients with patellofemoral (anterior knee pain) syndromes

Contraindications: Significant dynamic activity to lower extremities

Pearls of performance: When initially learning this exercise, the individual may need to be spotted or to have a handrail close by to maintain balance.

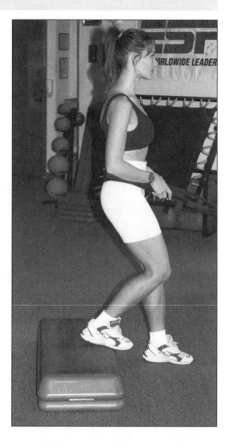

Lateral Step-Up

Start position: Standing with left or right side facing the steps

Exercise action: Step up sideways.

Purpose: To strengthen the lower extremity, to increase balance

Primary muscles used: Hip flexors, hip ab/adductors, quadriceps, hip extensors

Indications: To strengthen lower-extremity muscles, patients with ACL reconstructions, patients with patellofemoral (anterior knee pain) syndromes

Contraindications: Significant dynamic activity to lower extremities

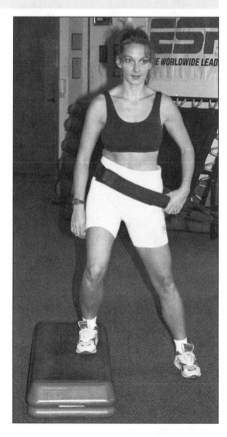

Standing Terminal Knee Extension With Rubber Tubing (Don Tigney, PT, Exercise)

Start position: Standing facing attachment of surgical tubing, with the tubing attached to a piece of equipment, a door, or other sturdy object

Exercise action: Flex the knee about 30° and then fully extend the knee; the tubing provides resistance to the extension of the knee in a closed chain position.

Purpose: To gain dynamic control over terminal extension of the knee in a weight-bearing position

Primary muscles used: Hip extensors, hamstrings, quadriceps, gastrocnemius

Indications: Individuals who have difficulty in performing active terminal extension of the knee; to prevent a quadriceps "lag"; to help a patient prepare the lower extremity, particularly the knee, for the demands of gait

Contraindications: When terminal knee extension is not desired due to a surgical procedure, soft-tissue healing constraints, and so on

Pearls of performance: Excellent exercise to help patients with knee-extension deficits and to prepare the knee for the demands of functional gait

Quadriceps lag is the presence of several degrees of knee flexion during the initial execution of a straight-leg raise exercise, indicating weakness or insufficiency of the quadriceps mechanism near full knee extension.

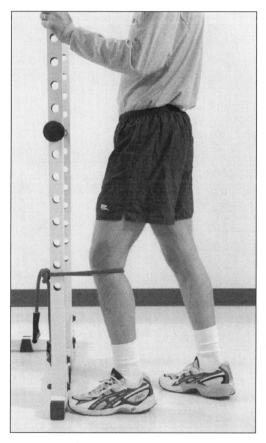
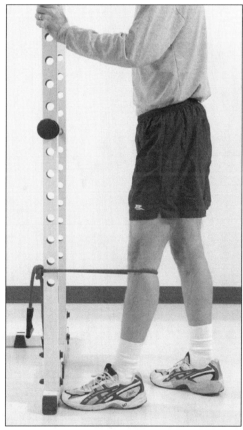

Elliptical Running Machine

Start position: Standing

Exercise action: Lower-extremity bilateral reciprocal endurance exercise

Purpose: To develop lower-extremity muscular endurance and cardiovascular endurance

Primary muscles used: Hip extensors, hamstrings, quadriceps, gastrocnemius

Indications: Individuals who have difficulty in performing active terminal extension of the knee; to prevent a quadriceps "lag"; to help a patient prepare the lower extremity, particularly the knee, for the demands of gait

Contraindications: When terminal knee extension is not desired due to a surgical procedure, soft-tissue healing constraints, and so on

Pearls of performance: This is a nonimpact, loaded, reciprocal exercise. Elliptical running machines most closely replicate the motion of running of any exercise equipment on the market.

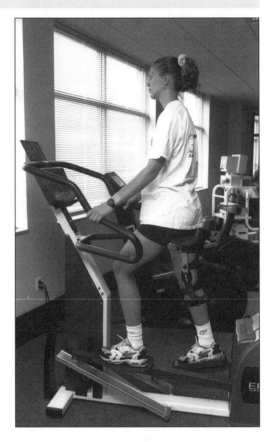

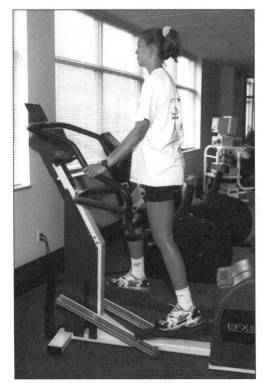

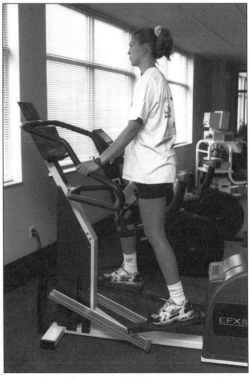

Lateral Bounding

Start position: Standing

Exercise action: Frontal plane movements with a bounding (power) movement

Purpose: To develop power in frontal-plane movements

Primary muscles used: Hip abductors, hip adductors, hip extensors, quadriceps, gastrocnemius

Contraindications: Collateral ligament injuries

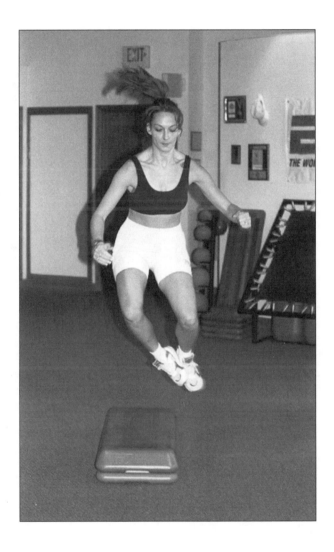

Side-Shuffle Agility Drills

Start position: Standing

Exercise action: Side-to-side movement of the feet in the frontal plane

Purpose: To develop neuromuscular quickness in the frontal plane

Primary muscles used: Hip abductors, hip adductors, quadriceps, gluteals, gastrocnemius, hamstrings

Contraindications: Collateral ligament injuries

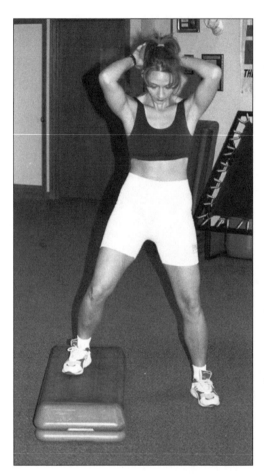
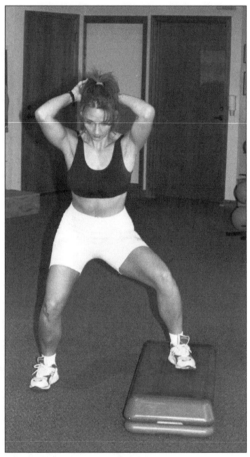

Carioca Agility Drills

Start position: Standing

Exercise action: Braiding or cross-stepping movement patterns

Purpose: To develop lateral movements with a crossover step

Primary muscles used: Hip abductors, hip adductors, quadriceps

Figure-Eight Agility Drills

Start position: Standing

Exercise action: Run in a figure-eight pattern.

Purpose: To develop ability to run in a circular format

Primary muscles used: All lower-extremity muscles

Indications: To develop multiple movements

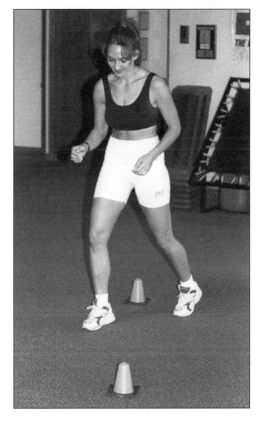

Cutting Drills

Start position: Standing

Exercise action: Plant the outside foot and make the appropriate angle cuts (30°, 45°, 60°, 90°), or crossover cuts by planting the inside foot.

Purpose: To develop the ability to turn sharply

Primary muscles used: All lower-extremity muscles

Contraindications: Unstable knees

Pearls of performance: This exercise can be performed with increasing intensity to increase the difficulty.

Depth Jumps

Start position: Standing on an object, such as a plyometric box

Exercise action: Jump down from the box to produce the stretch–shorten cycle.

Purpose: To develop power of the lower extremities

Primary muscles used: Quadriceps (eccentric muscle action), hip extensors

Contraindications: Unstable knees, lower-extremity joint chondrosis

Pearls of performance: This is the classic exercise that plyometrics evolved from.

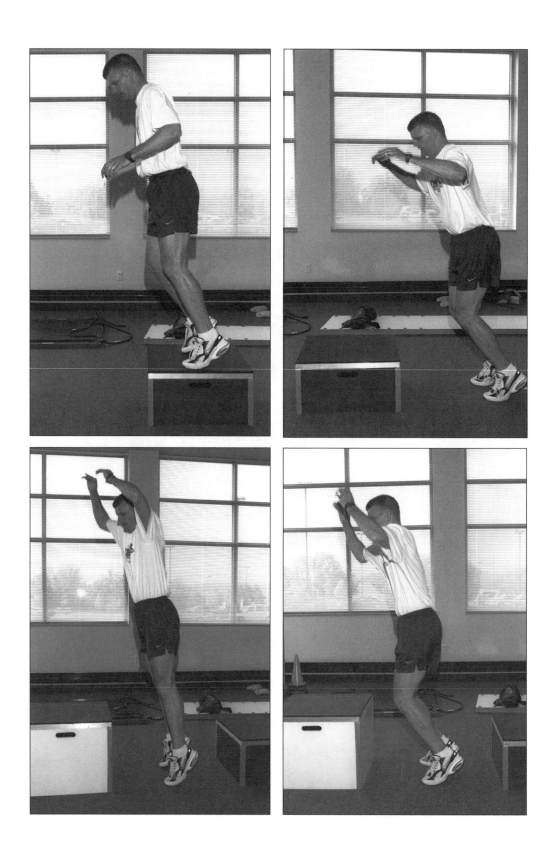

Balance Exercises, Two-Leg and One-Leg

Start position: Standing in a partially to fully weight-bearing position

Exercise action: Maintain balance

Purpose: To develop kinesthesia/proprioception

Primary muscles used: Quadriceps (eccentric muscle action), hip extensors, lower-extremity co-contractions

Contraindications: Unstable knees

Pearls of performance: Numerous variations of these exercises can be used, such as:
1. Partial to full weight bearing
2. Double-leg to single-leg exercises
3. Single-plane to multiplane balance boards

Tubing Walk

Start position: Stand with feet shoulder-width apart with Theraband tied around both legs in giant loop

Exercise action: With knees slightly flexed, step forward with one foot at a diagonal; alternate feet

Purpose: to develop general lower-extremity strength and balance

Primary muscles used: All lower-extremity muscle groups

Indication: Individuals with lower-extremity weakness and core stabilization training

Contraindications: Not for use in post-operative non-weight-bearing situations

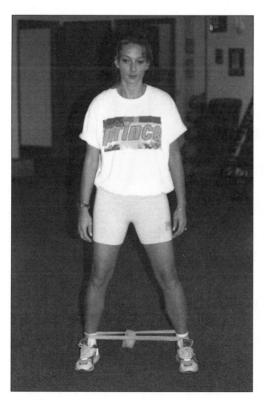 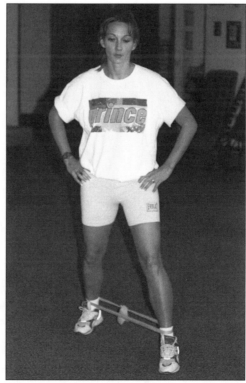

8

Upper-Extremity Closed Kinetic Chain Exercises

This chapter contains a series of closed kinetic chain exercises for the upper extremities that can be used for both rehabilitation and performance enhancement. The exercises are presented generally from simplest or most basic to more complex and difficult. The exercises presented early in this chapter are particularly suitable for individuals with shoulder pain or postoperative patients in rehabilitation. A thorough evaluation must be performed to determine whether these exercises are appropriate for the individual. Additionally, careful monitoring of an individual's signs and symptoms is important in determining progression of these exercises.

Figure 8.1 presents a chart useful in determining the volume or repetitions for resistive exercise training that is applicable to closed kinetic chain exercise (Fleck and Kraemer 1987). Sets with a higher number of repetitions (12 to 18 repetitions per set) have been recommended to improve local muscular endurance (Fleck and Kraemer 1987) and used by the authors of this text specifically for rehabilitation and in various stages of performance-enhancement training. Research clearly identifying the optimal number of sets, repetitions, and intensity of upper-extremity closed kinetic chain training is lacking. Exercise prescription is currently guided by extrapolating accepted research generated in open kinetic chain upper-extremity environments (Davies 1992; Fleck and Kramer 1987).

Each exercise for the upper extremity will be presented in the same fashion as in chapter 7 with exercise name, start position, exercise action, purpose, primary muscles used, indications, contraindications, and pearls of performance listed where indicated.

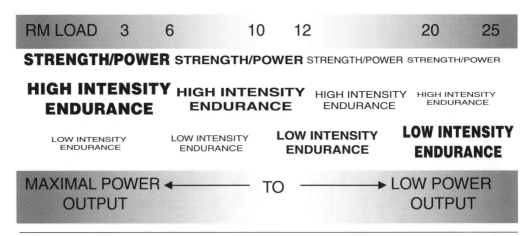

Figure 8.1 Theoretical repetition maximum (RM) continuum. RM load means the maximum number of properly executed repetitions that can be performed continuously with a given load. The goal of using different RM loading schemes is shown below the RM load.

Reprinted from Fleck and Kraemer 1987.

Weight-Bearing and Joint Approximation Exercises

Joint Approximation With Swiss Ball

Start position: Standing with slight trunk flexion with hand directly on Swiss ball or handle board to allow a more neutral wrist position

Exercise action: Press downward into the ball, "dimpling" the ball slightly (pressure can vary on intensity of exercise) while moving it in clockwise and counterclockwise circles of various sizes.

Purpose: Used early in training or rehabilitation to produce co-contraction of the scapular musculature, rotator cuff, and distal arm muscles

Primary muscles used: Serratus, trapezius, latissimus dorsi, rotator cuff, and triceps

Indications: Postoperatively and early in rehabilitation and training

Contraindications: Labral pathology and status/post acromioplasty where pressure or approximation of the humeral head is painful, acute rotator cuff tendinosis or bursitis

Pearls of performance: Exercise can be varied for home use by placing a basketball or standard-size playground ball on the seat of the chair. This exercise, an alternative to Codman's exercise for individuals with anterior instability, eliminates the anterior pressure typically encountered during an unsupported Codman's exercise. Virtually any direction, including diagonals, can be used in this exercise.

An advanced version of this exercise for performance enhancement places the individual in the prone position on a table, hanging off from the waist upward. One arm is supported on a Swiss ball while it makes small clockwise and counterclockwise circles. An additional variation of this exercise requires stabilization of the weight-bearing shoulder in the "plus" position to increase the recruitment of the serratus anterior (Moseley et al. 1992).

Rocker Board

Start position: Standing with hands on a rocker board placed approximately at waist level on a table or countertop

Exercise action: While leaning forward and bearing weight up through the shoulders, perform a side-to-side, front-to-back, or circular movements.

Purpose: Early exercise used to produce muscular co-contraction and begin to increase weight-bearing tolerance for the upper extremities

Primary muscles used: Serratus, trapezius, latissimus dorsi, rotator cuff, and triceps

Indications: Excellent early exercise in rehabilitation for producing joint approximation in and weight bearing by the upper extremities. Kibler et al. (1995) measured EMG activity during this exercise and reported a low output from the scapular stabilizers, rotator cuff, and deltoids (see table 6.2, p. 50).

Contraindications: Labral pathology and status/post acromioplasty where pressure or approximation of the humeral head is painful, acute rotator cuff tendinosis or bursitis

Wax On, Wax Off

Start position: On hands and knees, head in neutral position looking downward, and hands shoulder-width apart

Exercise action: With socks or slide-board boots worn on the hands, perform clockwise and counterclockwise circular motions unilaterally while the contralateral upper extremity stabilizes. Repeat on the other side. Activity can also be performed by moving both arms simultaneously.

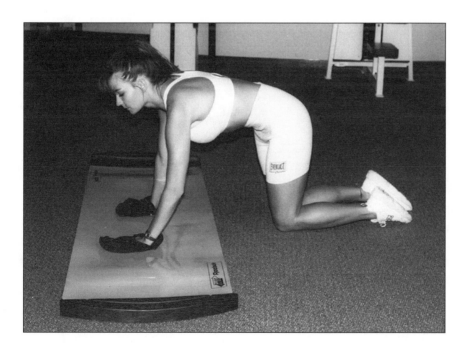

Purpose: To produce co-contraction of the muscles of the upper extremities, particularly the upper extremity that is bearing weight or stabilizing, not necessarily the extremity making the movements, and a functional movement pattern and position used in ADLs and in positional transition from the floor or ground. Weight bearing on the upper extremity promotes dynamic neuromuscular control and kinesthesia.

Primary muscles used: Serratus, trapezius, latissimus dorsi, rotator cuff, triceps, and deltoids

Indications: An endurance exercise for any shoulder pathology that needs enhanced scapular stabilization

Contraindications: Labral pathology and status/post acromioplasty where pressure or approximation of the humeral head is painful, acute rotator cuff tendinosis or bursitis

Pearls of performance: In the clinical or gym setting, a slide board and booties work well. For home use, socks on the hands and a tile floor are sufficient.

Modified Quadruped Rhythmic Stabilization (Perturbation Training)

Start position: On hands and knees on a table or floor, with the hands and knees directly under the shoulders and hips, respectively. The hands and knees are about shoulder-width apart. The head and spine are in a neutral position.

Exercise action: A partner, therapist, or trainer tells the individual, "Hold, don't let me move you," and performs short, rapid, pushing motions from side to side, front to back, and along diagonals, initially using a nonrandom pattern and progressing to a random pattern as stability and familiarity with the exercise develop. The pushing motions also progress from submaximal to maximal intensities and from slow to very fast.

Purpose: To increase upper-body strength and scapular and trunk stabilization

Primary muscles used: Serratus, trapezius, latissimus dorsi, rotator cuff, and triceps, but with added emphasis on the abdominals and back extensors (core stability), lower-extremity musculature, and deltoids

Indications: An endurance exercise for any shoulder pathology that needs enhanced scapular stabilization

Contraindications: Labral pathology and status/post acromioplasty where pressure or approximation of the humeral head is painful, acute rotator cuff tendinosis or bursitis, and posterior glenohumeral joint instability

Pearls of performance: The short, rapid, pushing motions produce brief periods of muscular stabilization and both concentric and eccentric muscular activation of the scapular stabilizers. The rhythmic stabilization typically applied in physical medicine uses slow pressure, with constant hand contact on the individual (Sullivan et al. 1982). The authors of this book find this rapid method clinically effective; the multidirectional manual pressures provide an element of proprioceptive challenge in addition to the more rapid recruitment of muscles. Furthermore, many functional activities require the more rapid neuromuscular reactive patterns facilitated with this exercise.

Push-Up Variations

Push-Up With a Plus

Start position: Standard push-up position with feet approximately shoulder-width apart, head and spine in neutral position

Exercise action: Lower body toward the floor only approximately half the distance of a standard push-up, then reverse direction and press forcibly outward, rounding the back like a cat and protracting the scapulas maximally.

Purpose: Permits a safe excursion for the glenohumeral joint and optimally recruits the scapular stabilizers.

Primary muscles used: Serratus anterior, pectoralis major and minor, triceps, rotator cuff, trapezius, abdominals, trunk extensors (core stabilization), and deltoids

Indications: Particularly applicable for any individual with scapular winging or a lack of scapular stability and for throwing athletes due to protection of the anterior shoulder capsule by the shortened range of motion on the lowering phase

Contraindications: Any anterior shoulder pain signals discontinuation of this exercise or any variation; posterior shoulder instabilities and labral lesions.

Pearls of performance: The individual can begin this exercise off the knees in the start position rather than off the toes. This decreases the load on the shoulder significantly. The individual can progress to standard push-up position when more optimal muscular recruitment and scapular stabilization is present. Additionally, lowering the body only a third of the way down may decrease discomfort for individuals who have shoulder pathology or a history of shoulder pathology. Research has clearly validated the plus position (Moseley et al. 1992).

Plyometric Wall Push-Up

Start position: Standing with feet shoulder-width apart, arms held directly out in front of the body at 90° of elevation against the wall. Feet are approximately 2 to 3 ft (0.6–0.9 m) away from the wall.

Exercise action: The chest is lowered toward the wall until the elbows are bent approximately 45° to 60°. The individual then forcefully pushes from the wall so that the hands leave the wall and the body stands upright. The body again is lowered to the wall, where the upper extremities eccentrically absorb the force of body weight.

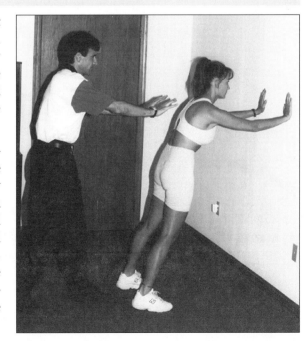

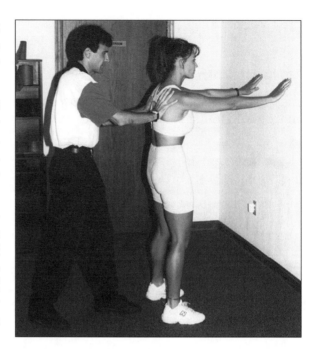

Purpose: The body does not work completely against gravity as in the standard push-up or push-up with a plus.

Primary muscles used: Serratus anterior, pectoralis major and minor, deltoids, triceps, rotator cuff, trapezius, abdominals, and trunk extensors (core stabilization)

Indications: Particularly applicable for any individual with scapular winging or a lack of scapular stability and for throwing athletes due to protection of the anterior shoulder capsule by the shortened range of motion on the lowering phase

Contraindications: None typically, but any anterior shoulder pain signals discontinuation of this exercise or any variation; posterior glenohumeral joint instability and labral pathology.

Pearls of performance: Emphasize scapular protraction during the forceful push-off phase of this exercise to improve recruitment of the serratus anterior muscle. A partner can be used to provide a pushing motion to increase the force absorption required and to provide a plyometric-like environment during this exercise.

Press-Up

Start position: Seated in a chair or on a table or countertop

Exercise action: Keeping the hips flexed at a 90° angle and shoulders back, press down onto the chair or tabletop, lifting the buttocks off the surface. Slowly return to the start position.

Purpose: To work the shoulder girdle depressors

Primary muscles used: Pectoralis minor, triceps, rhomboids, lower trapezius, latissimus dorsi, serratus anterior, abdominals, and back extensors

Indications: Scapular winging and general upper-body strengthening

Contraindications: Acute phase rotator cuff and bursal pathology; AC joint injury; status/post acromioplasty; or status/post superior labrum, anterior and posterior (SLAP) repair due to possibility of superior migration of the humeral head during exercise if adequate glenohumeral compression and dynamic stability are not present

Pearls of performance: Scapular muscle activity measured by Moseley et al. (1992) was low during this exercise, but many functional activities require shoulder depression and stabilization. Small blocks can be placed under the hands to increase the range of motion. Caution should be used when adding blocks since too much height stresses the anterior capsule of the shoulder and may be inappropriate, particularly for overhead athletes and persons with anterior shoulder instability.

Wheelbarrow Walks

Start position: In standard push-up position with hands directly under shoulders and approximately shoulder-width apart

Exercise action: A partner, therapist, or trainer grasps the feet of the individual, who takes small, controlled "steps" with the hands. The individual moves in different directions, including front to back, side to side, and carioca-type side shuffling.

Purpose: Scapular stabilization, general upper-body conditioning, and balance

Primary muscles used: Serratus anterior, pectoralis major and minor, triceps, rotator cuff, deltoids, trapezius, abdominals, and trunk extensors (core stabilization)

Indications: Scapular winging and general upper-body strengthening

Contraindications: Acute phase rotator cuff pathology, status/post acromioplasty or status/post SLAP repair due to possibility of superior migration of the humeral head during exercise if adequate glenohumeral compression and dynamic stability are not present; posterior glenohumeral joint instability

Pearls of performance: To substitute for a partner, a stair-climbing machine can be used. Start with the feet on the ground shoulder-width apart. Perform stepping-type motions with the upper extremities in an alternating pattern.

Upper-Body Treadmill Walking

Start position: On hands and knees perpendicular to the side of a treadmill, with the hands on the center of the treadmill band and knees directly under the hips

Exercise action: Using a slow, controlled treadmill speed with no incline, the hands are walked sideways using a cross-hand technique.

Purpose: To alternately bear weight on the upper extremities for general upper-body strengthening and scapular stabilization

Primary muscles used: Serratus anterior, pectoralis major and minor, triceps, rotator cuff, deltoids, trapezius, abdominals, and trunk extensors (core stabilization)

Indications: Intermediate weight-bearing exercise progression for shoulder rehabilitation and general strengthening

Contraindications: Acute phase rotator cuff pathology, status/post acromioplasty or status/post SLAP repair due to possibility of superior migration of the humeral head during exercise if adequate glenohumeral compression and dynamic stability are not present; posterior glenohumeral joint instability

Pearls of performance: Variations include carioca (over then under crossover walking) and progressing from the hands-and-knees position to a standard push-up position off the toes.

Isokinetic Protraction and Retraction

Start position: Seated with shoulder elevated 90° in the scapular plane. Stabilization must be provided to minimize trunk and elbow motion.

Exercise action: Perform a small protraction and retraction motion with the shoulder in 90° of elevation in the scapular plane. Due to the small arc of motion inherent in true scapular protraction and retraction, slower isokinetic training velocities should be used (e.g., 30°, 60°, 90°, and 120° per second).

Purpose: To strengthen the scapular protractors and retractors

Primary muscles used: Serratus anterior, rhomboids, trapezius

Indications: Individuals with scapular winging and shoulder weakness

Contraindications: None

Pearls of performance: Davies and Dickhoff-Hoffman (1993) published normative data on scapular protraction and retraction from 125 shoulders. They reported an approximate 1:1 ratio of protraction and retraction strength. Use of the isokinetic dynamometer for this movement pattern allows objective testing of scapular muscle strength.

Step-Up Variations

Upper-Extremity Step-Up

Start position: On hands and knees (beginning level), with hands and knees directly under shoulders and hips, respectively, and hands shoulder-width apart. A 6- to 8-in. (15–20 cm) step or structure is placed to one side of the individual.

Exercise action: Place one hand on the step. Extend the elbow in a pressing up movement. Place the other hand on top of the hand already on the step while performing a plus maneuver by maximally protracting or rounding the shoulders outward. Move the hands in reverse order back to the ground.

Purpose: General upper-body strengthening; particularly useful for scapular stabilization

Primary muscles used: Serratus anterior, trapezius, rotator cuff, deltoids, pectorals, latissimus dorsi, and triceps

Indications: Individuals with upper-body weakness and scapular winging

Contraindications: Posterior glenohumeral joint instability; labral pathology

Pearls of performance: This exercise is initially started in the hands-and-knees position and progresses to the standard "on toes" push-up start position. Addition of the plus movement of the scapulas increases serratus anterior activation (Moseley et al. 1992).

Variation 1: Rather than pushing up onto a stable platform, a medicine ball can be used, which creates instability and forces the individual to stabilize in all directions over the ball.

Variation 2: Any upper-arm step-up exercises performed off the toes in the push-up position can be made more challenging by placing the feet on a 6- to 8-in. (15- to 20-cm) platform or a chair.

Balance Progression Exercises

Quadruped on Balance Board

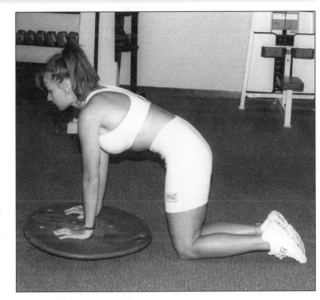

Start position: On hands and knees, with hands and knees directly under shoulders and hips, respectively, and hands approximately shoulder-width apart on a balance or rocker board

Exercise action: In the early stages of rehabilitation, the individual simply attempts to balance over the board, keeping all sides of the board off the ground. In later stages, the board is moved in a circular pattern both clockwise and counterclockwise, keeping all edges of the board off the ground.

Purpose: General upper-body strengthening and proprioceptive training for the upper body and trunk

Primary muscles used: Serratus anterior, trapezius, rotator cuff, deltoids, pectorals, latissimus dorsi, triceps, wrist and finger flexors

Indications: For upper-extremity weakness or loss of scapular control or to initiate weight bearing in the upper extremities following injury or surgery

Contraindications: Posterior glenohumeral joint instability and labral pathology

Pearls of performance: The individual can alternate between static holds of the scapular protraction, "plus" position, and retraction while performing the circular movement patterns and can move from full protraction to retraction while balancing. The size of the ball placed under the board can be manipulated to make the exercise more or less challenging.

Push-Up With a Plus on Balance Board

Start position: Standard push-up position with hands shoulder-width apart on a balance board. The individual maintains the plus position by maximally protracting the shoulders during the exercise.

Exercise action: Balance on the board, or perform clockwise and counterclockwise circular movements with the board.

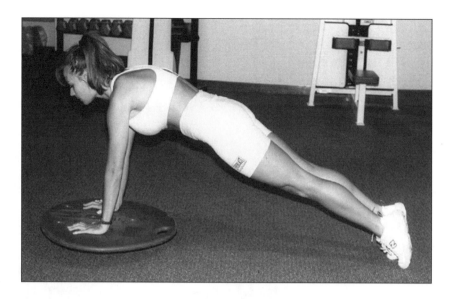

Purpose: General upper-body strengthening and proprioceptive training for the upper body and trunk

Primary muscles used: Serratus anterior, trapezius, rotator cuff, deltoids, pectorals, latissimus dorsi, triceps, wrist and finger flexors

Indications: For upper-extremity weakness or loss of scapular control or to initiate weight bearing in the upper extremities following injury or surgery

Contraindications: Patients lacking core stability

Pearls of performance: During muscular fatigue the medial borders of the scapulas often become more prominent, so careful monitoring of scapular position during the exercise gives an objective guide for the length of balancing and number of sets.

Swiss Ball and Balance Board

Start position: Legs are placed over Swiss ball at approximately the midtibial level. Hands are placed shoulder-width apart on a balance board.

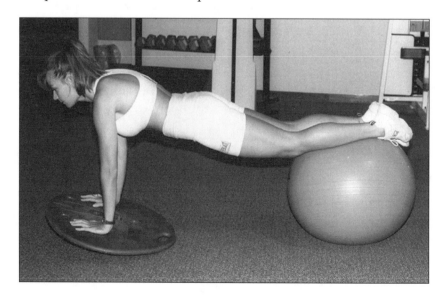

Exercise action: Balance on the board, or perform clockwise and counterclockwise circular movements with the board.

Purpose: General upper-body strengthening and proprioceptive training for the upper body and trunk

Primary muscles used: Serratus anterior, trapezius, rotator cuff, deltoids, pectorals, latissimus dorsi, triceps, wrist and finger flexors

Indications: For upper-extremity weakness or loss of scapular control or to initiate weight bearing in the upper extremities following injury or surgery

Contraindications: Posterior glenohumeral joint instability and labral pathology

Pearls of performance: Manipulating the size of the ball and the position of the ball against the body can increase or decrease the difficulty of this exercise. Additionally, the plus position can increase serratus anterior activation (Moseley et al. 1992).

Cuff Link Balancing (Bilateral and Unilateral)

Start position: Standard push-up position with feet approximately shoulder-width apart and hands grasping the handles of the Cuff Link device

Exercise action: Static or dynamic balance on the Cuff Link and/or performed clockwise and counterclockwise circular movements with the device.

Purpose: General upper-body strengthening and proprioceptive training for the upper body and trunk

Primary muscles used: Serratus anterior, trapezius, rotator cuff, deltoids, pectorals, latissimus dorsi, triceps, wrist and finger flexors

Indications: For upper-extremity weakness or loss of scapular control or to initiate weight bearing in the upper extremities following injury or surgery

Contraindications: Posterior glenohumeral joint instability and labral pathology

Pearls of performance: Unilateral exercise can be performed by changing to a central handle position as pictured on page 98.

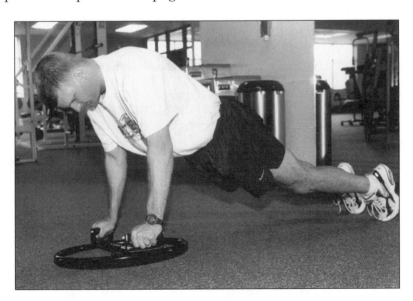

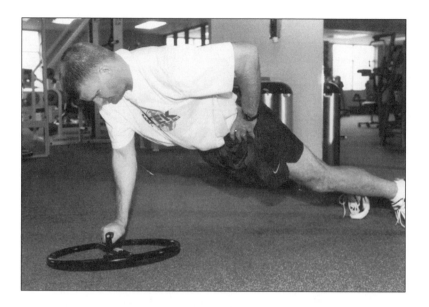

Tri-ped Rhythmic Stabilization

Start position: On hands and knees placed directly under the shoulders and hips respectively. The hands are placed approximately shoulder-width apart.

Exercise action: A partner grasps the non-exercising (in patients, uninjured) extremity in a standard handshake grasp. The shoulder and elbow of this arm are to remain fixed in 90° of shoulder flexion and elbow flexion. The partner alternately pushes and pulls the non-exercising hand as the individual attempts to keep stable and remain as stationary as possible. The resistance can be applied from side to side and diagonally as well. Of particular importance is the individual's ability to remain stable during the transition from one direction to another.

Purpose: Scapular stabilization and proprioceptive training for the upper body and trunk (core stability)

Primary muscles used: Serratus anterior, trapezius, rotator cuff, deltoids, pectorals, latissimus dorsi, triceps, wrist and finger flexors

Indications: For upper-extremity weakness or loss of scapular control or to initiate weight bearing in the upper extremities following injury or surgery

Contraindications: Individuals with posterior glenohumeral joint instability, lacking core stability

Pearls of performance: Monitoring the medial and inferior borders of the scapula is an excellent objective marker for muscular fatigue and for setting work–rest cycles and the duration of exercise.

References

Andersen SB, Terwilliger DM, Denegar CR. 1995. Comparison of open versus closed kinetic chain test positions for measuring joint position sense. J Sport Rehabil 4:165–171.

Anderson, MA. 1989. The relationship among isometric, isotonic, and isokinetic concentric and eccentric quadriceps and hamstring force and three components of athletic performance. Ann Arbor, MI: University Microfilm International.

Anderson, MA, Gieck JH, Perrin D, et al. 1991. The relationship among isometric, isotonic and isokinetic concentric and eccentric quadriceps and hamstring force and three components of athletic performance. J Orthop Sports Phys Ther 14(3):114–120.

Augustsson J, Esko A, Thomee R, Svantesson U. 1998. Weight training of the thigh muscles using closed vs. open kinetic chain exercises: a comparison of performance enhancement. J Orthop Sports Phys Ther 27(1):3–8.

Aune AK, Cawley PW, Ekeland A. 1997. Quadriceps muscle contraction protects the anterior cruciate ligament during anterior tibial translation. Am J Sports Med 25(2):187–195.

Ballantyne BT, O'Hare SJ, Paschall JL, Pavia-Smith MM, Pitz AM, Gillon JF, Soderberg GL. 1993. Electromyographic activity of selected shoulder muscles in commonly used therapeutic exercises. Phys Ther 73(10):668–682.

Barber SD, Noyes FR, Mangine RE, McCloskey JW, Hartman W. 1990. Quantitative assessment of functional limitations in normal and anterior cruciate ligament deficient knees. Clin Orthop 255:204–214.

Beynnon BD, Fleming BC, Johnson RJ, Nichols CE, Renstrom PA, Pope MH. 1995. Anterior cruciate ligament strain behavior during rehabilitation exercises in vivo. Am J Sports Med 23(1):24–34.

Beynnon BD, Johnson RJ, Fleming BC, Renstrom PA, Nichols CE, Pope MH, Haugh LD. 1994. The measurement of elongation of anterior cruciate ligament grafts in vivo. J Bone Joint Surg Am 76(4):520–531.

Beynnon BD, Johnson RJ, Fleming BC, Stankewich CJ, Renstrom PA, Nichols CE. 1997. The strain behavior of the anterior cruciate ligament during squatting and active flexion-extension: a comparison of open and closed kinetic chain exercise. Am J Sports Med 25(6):823–829.

Blackard DO, Jensen RL, Ebben WP. 1999. Use of EMG analysis in challenging kinetic chain terminology. Med Sci Sports Exerc 31(3):443–448.

Blackburn TA, McLeod WD, White B, Wofford L. 1990. EMG analysis of the posterior rotator cuff exercises. J Athl Training 25:40–45.

Bolz S, Davies GJ. 1984. Leg length differences and correlation with total leg strength. J Orthop Sports Phys Ther 6:123–129.

Buckley J. 1997 Aug 6. Closed kinetic chain—an open or shut case? Frontline:8–9.

Buckley JP, Kerwin DG. 1988. The role of the biceps and triceps brachii during tennis serving. Ergonomics 31(11):1621–1629.

Bullock-Saxton JE. 1994. Local sensation changes and altered hip muscle function following severe ankle sprain. Phys Ther 74(1):17–23.

Bunn J. 1972. Scientific principles of coaching. Englewood Cliffs, NJ: Prentice Hall.

Bynum EB, Barrack RL, Alexander AH. 1995. Open versus closed chain kinetic exercises after anterior cruciate ligament reconstruction: a prospective randomized study. Am J Sports Med 23(4):401–406.

Chen SK, Simonion PT, Wickiewicz TL, Warren RF. 1999. Radiographic evaluation of glenohumeral kinematics: a muscle fatigue model. J Shoulder Elbow Surg 8:49–52.

Codman EA. 1934. The shoulder. 2nd ed. Boston: Thomas Todd.

Cook TM, Zimmerman CL, Lux KM, Neubrand CM, Nicholson TD. 1992. EMG comparison of lateral step-up and stepping machine exercise. J Orthop Sports Phys Ther 16(3):108–113.

Daniels L, Worthingham C. 1986. Muscle testing: techniques of manual examination. 5th ed. Philadelphia: Saunders.

Davies GJ. 1992. A compendium of isokinetics in clinical usage. LaCrosse, WI: S & S.

Davies GJ. 1995a. Descriptive study comparing open kinetic chain and closed kinetic chain isokinetic testing of the lower extremity in 200 patients with selected knee injuries [abstract]. In: Proceedings 12th International Congress–World Confederation for Physical Therapy; Washington, DC: American Physical Therapy Association. p. 906.

Davies GJ. 1995b. The need for critical thinking in rehabilitation. J Sport Rehabil 4:1–22.

Davies GJ, Dickoff-Hoffman S. 1993. Neuromuscular testing and rehabilitation of the shoulder complex. J Orthop Sports Phys Ther 18(2):449–458.

Davies GJ, Ellenbecker TS. 1993. Scientific and clinical rationale for utilization of a total arm strength rehabilitation program for shoulder and elbow overuse injuries. APTA Orthopaedic Section, Home Study Course, LaCrosse, WI.

Davies GJ, Ellenbecker TS. 1998. Application of isokinetics in testing and rehabilitation. In: Andrews JR, Harrelson GL, Wilk KE, editors. Physical rehabilitation of the injured athlete. 2nd ed. Philadelphia: Saunders. p. 219–259.

Davies GJ, Heiderscheit BC. 1997. Reliability of the Lido Linea Closed Kinetic Chain Isokinetic Dynamometer. J Orthop Sports Phys Ther 25(2):133–136.

Davies GJ, Heiderscheit BC, Clark M. 1995. Open kinetic chain assessment and rehabilitation. Athl Training Sports Health Care Perspect 1:347–370.

Davies GJ, Heiderscheit BC, Clark M. 2000. The scientific and clinical rationale for the use of open and closed kinetic chain rehabilitation. In: Ellenbecker TS, editor. Knee ligament rehabilitation. 2nd ed. Philadelphia: Churchill Livingstone. p. 291–300.

Davies GJ, Heiderscheit BC, Schulte R, Manske R, Neitzel J. 2000. The scientific and clinical rationale for the integrated approach to open and closed kinetic chain rehabilitation. Orthop Phys Ther Clin North Am 9(2):247–267.

Davies GJ, Wilk K, Ellenbecker TS. 1997. Assessment of strength. In: Malone TR, McPoil TG, Nitz AJ, editors. Orthopaedic and sports physical therapy. 3rd ed. St. Louis: Mosby-Year Book. p. 225–257.

Davies GJ, Zillmer DA. 2000. Functional progression of exercise during rehabilitation. In: Ellenbecker TS, editor. Knee ligament rehabilitation. 2nd ed. Philadelphia: Churchill Livingstone.

Decker MJ, Hintermeister RA, Faber KJ, Hawkins RJ. 1999. Serratus anterior muscle activity during selected rehabilitation exercises. Am J Sports Med 27(6):784–791.

Delitto A, Irrgang JJ, Harner DC, Fu FH, Nessi S. 1993. Relationship of isokinetic quadriceps peak torque and work to one legged hop and vertical jump in ACL reconstructed knees. Phys Ther 73(6):S85.

DiFabio RP. 1999. Making jargon from kinetic and kinematic chains. J Orthop Sports Phys Ther 29(3):142–143.

DiGiovine NM, Jobe FW, Pink M, Perry J. 1994. An electromyographic analysis of the upper extremity in pitching. J Shoulder Elbow Surg 1:15–25.

Dillman CJ. 1991. [Presentation on the upper extremity in tennis and throwing athletes.] United States Tennis Association National Meeting, March, Tucson, AZ.

Dillman CJ, Murray TA, Hintermeister RA. 1994. Biomechanical differences of open and closed kinetic chain exercises with respect to the shoulder. J Sport Rehabil 3:228–238.

Donkers MJ, An KN, Chao EY, Morrey BF. 1993. Hand position affects elbow load during push-up exercise. J Biomech 26:625–632.

Doody SG, Freedman L, Waterland JC. 1970. Shoulder movements during abduction in the scapular plane. Arch Phys Med Rehabil 51(10):595–604.

Doucette SA, Child DD. 1996. The effect of open and closed chain exercise and knee joint position on patellar tracking in lateral patellar compression syndrome. J Orthop Sports Phys Ther 23(2):104–110.

Draganich LF, Jaeger RJ, Knalj AR. 1989. Coactivation of the hamstrings and quadriceps during extension of the knee. J Bone Joint Surg Am 71(7):1075–1081.

Dvir Z. 1996. An isokinetic study of combined activity of the hip and knee extensors. Clin Biomech 11(3):135–138.

Ellenbecker TS. 1991. A total arm strength profile of highly skilled tennis players. Isokinet Exerc Sci 1:9–21.

Ellenbecker TS. 1992. Shoulder internal and external rotation strength and range of motion of highly skilled junior tennis players. Isokinet Exerc Sci 2:1–8.

Ellenbecker TS, Cappel K. 2000. Clinical application of closed kinetic chain exercises in the upper extremities. Orthop Phys Ther Clin North Am 9(2):231–246.

Ellenbecker TS, Derscheid GL. 1989. Rehabilitation of overuse injuries of the shoulder. Clin Sports Med 8:583–604.

Ellenbecker TS, Mattalino AJ. 1997. Comparison of open and closed kinetic chain upper extremity tests in patients with rotator cuff pathology and glenohumeral joint instability [abstract]. J Orthop Sports Phys Ther 25(1):84.

Ellenbecker TS, Roetert EP. 1996. A bilateral comparison of upper extremity unilateral closed chain stance stability in elite junior tennis players and professional baseball pitchers [abstract]. Med Sci Sports Exerc 28(5):S105.

Ellenbecker TS, Selby LM, Roetert EP. 1999. Isokinetic profile of elbow flexion/extension strength in elite junior tennis players [abstract]. Med Sci Sports Exerc 31(5):S296.

Elliott BC, Marsh T, Blanksby B. 1986. A three dimensional cinematographic analysis of the tennis serve. Int J Sport Biomech 2:260–271.

Elliott BC, Marshall RN, Noffal GJ. 1995. Contributions to upper limb segment rotations during the power serve in tennis. J Appl Biomech 11(4):433–442.

Ernst GP, Saliba E, Diduch DR, Hurwitz SR, Ball DW. 2000. Lower extremity compensations following anterior cruciate ligament reconstruction. Phys Ther 80(3):251–260.

Escamilla RF, Fleisig GS, Zheng N, Barrentine SW, Wilk KE, Andrews JR. 1998. Biomechanics of the knee during closed kinetic chain and open kinetic chain exercises. Med Sci Sports Exerc 30(4):556–569.

Feiring DC, Ellenbecker TS. 1996. Single versus multiple joint isokinetic testing with ACL reconstructed patients. Isokinet Exerc Sci 6:109–115.

Feltner ME, Dapena J. 1986. Dynamics of the shoulder and elbow joints of the throwing arm during a baseball pitch. Int J Sport Biomech 2:235–259.

Fitzgerald GK. 1997. Open versus closed kinetic chain exercise: issues in rehabilitation after anterior cruciate ligament reconstructive surgery. Phys Ther 77:1747–1754.

Fitzgerald GK, Axe MJ, Snyder-Mackler L. 2000. The efficacy of perturbation training in nonoperative anterior cruciate ligament rehabilitation programs for physically active individuals. Phys Ther 80(2):128–140.

Fleck SJ, Kraemer WJ. 1987. Designing resistance training programs. Champaign, IL: Human Kinetics.

Fleisig GS, Andrews JR, Dillman CJ, Escamilla RF. 1995. Kinetics of baseball pitching with implications about injury mechanisms. Am J Sports Med 23(2):233–239.

Fleming BC, Beynnon BD, Renstrom PA, Johnson RJ, Nichols CE, Peura GD, Uh BS. 1999. The strain behavior of the anterior cruciate ligament during stair climbing: an in-vivo study. Arthroscopy 15(2):185–191.

Freidhoff G, Davies GJ, Malone T. 1998. Chain links: rehabilitation program should balance open and closed kinetic chain activities. Biomechanics 5:59–62, 66–69.

Gleim GW, Nicholas JA, Webb JN. 1978. Isokinetic evaluation following leg injuries. Physician Sports Med 6:74–82.

Goldbeck TG, Davies GJ. 2000. Test-retest reliability of the closed kinetic chain upper extremity stability test: a clinical field test. J Sport Rehabil 9:35–45.

Gowitzke BA, Millner S. 1988. Scientific bases of human movement. Baltimore: Williams & Wilkins.

Graham VL, Gehlson GM, Edwards JA. 1993. Electromyographic evaluation of closed and open kinetic chain knee rehabilitation exercises. J Athl Training 28(1):23–30.

Greenberger HB, Paterno MV. 1995. Relationship of knee extensor strength and hopping test performance in the assessment of lower extremity function. J Orthop Sports Phys Ther 22(5):202–206.

Groppel JL. 1992. High tech tennis. 2nd ed. Champaign, IL: Human Kinetics.

Hanavan EP. 1964. A mathematical model of the human body. Dayton, OH: Wright-Patterson Air Force Base. AMRL-TR-64-102.

Harryman DT, Sidles JA, Clark JM, McQuade KJ, Gibb TD, Matsen FA. 1990. Translation of the humeral head on the glenoid with passive glenohumeral motion. J Bone Joint Surg Am 72(9):1334–1343.

Henning CE, Lynch MA, Glick KR. 1985. An in vivo strain gauge study of elongation of the anterior cruciate ligament. Am J Sports Med 13(1):22–26.

Hintermeister RA, Lange GW, Schultheis JM, Bey MJ, Hawkins RJ. 1998. Electromyographic activity and applied load during shoulder rehabilitation exercises using elastic resistance. Am J Sports Med 26(2):210–220.

Hsieh HH, Walker PS. 1976. Stabilizing mechanisms of the loaded and unloaded knee joint. J Bone Joint Surg Am 58(1):87–93.

Hubley CS, Wells RP. 1983. A work-energy approach to determine individual joint contribution to vertical jump performance. Eur J Appl Physiol 50:247–254.

Inman VT, Saunders JB, Abbot LC. 1944. Observations on the function of the shoulder joint. J Bone Joint Surg Am 26A:1–30.

Isear JA Jr, Erickson JC, Worrell TW. 1997. EMG analysis of lower extremity muscle recruitment patterns during an unloaded squat. Med Sci Sports Exerc 29(4):532–539.

Johansson C, Lorentzon R, Fugl-Meyer AR. 1989. Isokinetic muscular performance of the quadriceps in elite ice hockey players. Am J Sports Med 17(1):30–34.

Jorgensen K. 1976. Force velocity relationships in human elbow flexors and extensors. In: Komi PV, editor. Biomechanics V. Baltimore: University Park Press. p. 145–151.

Kapandji IA. 1987. The physiology of the joints. Volume 2. London: Churchill Livingstone.

Kibler WB. 1991. The role of the scapula in the overhead throwing motion. Contemp Orthop 22:525–532.

Kibler WB. 1993. Evaluation of sports demands as a diagnostic tool in shoulder disorders. In: Matsen, FA, Fu FH, Hawkins RJ, editors. The shoulder: a balance of mobility and stability. Rosemont, IL: American Academy of Orthopaedic Surgeons.

Kibler WB. 1994. Clinical biomechanics of the elbow in tennis: implications for evaluation and diagnosis. Med Sci Sports Exerc 26(10):1203–1206.

Kibler WB. 1998a. The role of the scapula in athletic shoulder function. Am J Sports Med 26(2):325–337.

Kibler WB. 1998b. Shoulder rehabilitation: principles and practice. Med Sci Sports Exerc 30(4):S40–S50.

Kibler WB, Livingston B, Bruce R. 1995. Current concepts in shoulder rehabilitation. In: Advances in operative orthopaedics. Volume 3. St. Louis: Mosby-Year Book. p. 249–297.

Koenig JM, Jahn DM, Dohmeier TE, Cleland JW. 1995. The effect of bench step aerobics on muscular strength, power, and endurance. J Strength Conditioning Res 9(1):43–46.

Kulund DN, Rockwell DA, Brubaker CE. 1979. The long term effects of playing tennis. Physician Sports Med 7:87–92.

Lephart SM, Henry TJ. 1996. The physiological basis for open and closed kinetic chain rehabilitation for the upper extremity. J Sport Rehabil 5(1):71–87.

Lephart SM, Henry TJ, Riemann BL, Giannantonio FP, Fu FH. 1998. The effects of neuromuscular control exercises on functional stability in the unstable shoulder. J Athl Training 33(2):S15.

Litchfield DG, Jeno S, Mabey R. 1998. The lateral scapular slide test: is it valid in detecting glenohumeral impingement syndrome? [abstract]. Phys Ther 78(5):S29.

Loy SF, Conley LM, Sacco ER, Vincent WJ, Holland GJ, Sletten EG, Trueblood PR. 1994. Effects of stairclimbing on VO_2max and quadriceps strength in middle-aged females. Med Sci Sports Exerc 26(2):241–247.

Lutz GS, Palmitier RA, An KN, Chao, EY. 1993. Comparison of tibiofemoral joint forces during open kinetic chain and closed kinetic chain exercises. J Bone Joint Surg Am 75(5):732–739.

Lysholm M, Messner K. 1995. Sagittal plane translation of the tibia in anterior cruciate ligament deficient knees during commonly used rehabilitation exercises. Scand J Med Sci Sports 5:49–56.

Malanga FA, Jenp YN, Growney ES, An KN. 1996. EMG analysis of shoulder positioning in testing and strengthening the supraspinatus. Med Sci Sports Exerc 28(6):661–664.

Marshall RN, Elliott BC. 2000. Long-axis rotation: the missing link in proximal-to-distal segmental sequencing. J Sports Sci 18:247–254.

Marshall RN, Noffal GJ, Legnani G. 1993. Simulation of the tennis serve: factors affecting elbow torques related to medial epicondylitis. Paris: ISB.

Marshall RN, Wood GA. 1986. Movement expectation and simulations: segment interactions in drop punt kicking. In: Adrian M, Deutch H, editors. Biomechanics: the 1984 Olympic Scientific Congress Proceedings. Eugene, OR: Microform. p. 111–118.

McGee C, Kersting E, McLean K, Davies G. 1999. Standard rehabilitation vs. standard plus closed kinetic chain rehabilitation for patients with shoulder pathologies: a rehabilitation outcomes study [abstract]. Phys Ther 79(5):S65.

Miller JP, Sedory D, Croce RV. 1997a. Leg rotation and vastus medialis oblique/vastus lateralis electromyogram activity ratio during closed chain kinetic exercises prescribed for patellofemoral pain. J Athl Training 32(3):216–220.

Miller JP, Sedory D, Croce RV. 1997b. Vastus medialis obliquus and vastus lateralis activity in patients with and without patellofemoral pain syndrome. J Sport Rehabil 6:1–10.

More RC, Karras BT, Neiman R, Fritschy D, Woo SL, Daniel DM. 1993. Hamstrings—an anterior cruciate ligament protagonist: an in vitro study. Am J Sports Med 21(2):231–237.

Morrey BF, An KN. 1983. Articular and ligamentous contributions to stability of the elbow joint. Am J Sports Med 11:315.

Moseley JB, Jobe FW, Pink M, Perry J, Tibone J. 1992. EMG analysis of the scapular muscles during a shoulder rehabilitation program. Am J Sports Med 20(2):128–134.

Neer CS. 1983. Impingement lesions. Clin Orthop 173:70–77.

Neitzel JA, Davies GJ, Kernozek T, Fater DC. 2000. Closed kinetic chain weight bearing response following anterior cruciate ligament reconstruction [master's thesis]. LaCrosse: University of Wisconsin.

Nicholas JA, Strizak AM, Veras G. 1976. A study of thigh muscle weakness in different pathological states of the lower extremity. Am J Sports Med 4:241–248.

Ninos JC, Irrgang JJ, Burdett R, Weiss JR. 1997. Electromyographic analysis of the squat performed in self selected lower extremity neutral rotation and 30 degrees of lower extremity turn-out from the self selected neutral position. J Orthop Sports Phys Ther 25(5):307–315.

Noyes FR, Barber SD, Mangine RE. 1991. Abnormal lower limb symmetry determined by functional hop test after anterior cruciate ligament rupture. Am J Sports Med 19:513–518.

O'Brien SJ, Neves MC, Arnoczky SP, Rozbruck SR, Dicarlo EF, Warren RF, Schwartz R, Wickiewicz TL. 1990. The anatomy and histology of the inferior glenohumeral ligament complex of the shoulder. Am J Sports Med 18(5):449–456.

Ohkoshi Y, Yasuda K, Kaneda K, Wada T, Yamanaka M. 1991. Biomechanical analysis of rehabilitation in the standing position. Am J Sports Med 19(6):605–611.

Palmitier RA, An KN, Scott SG, Chao EY. 1991. Kinetic chain exercise in knee rehabilitation. Sports Med 11(6):402–413.

Plagenhoef S. 1971. Patterns of human motion. Englewood Cliffs, NJ: Prentice Hall.

Poppen NK, Walker PS. 1976. Normal and abnormal motion of the shoulder. J Bone Joint Surg Am 58(2):195–201.

Priest JD, Braden V, Gerberich SG. 1980. An analysis of players with and without pain. Physician Sports Med 8:81–91.

Priest JD, Nagel DA. 1976. Tennis shoulder. Am J Sports Med 4:28–42.

Putnam CA. 1993. Sequential motions of the body segments in striking and throwing skills: descriptions and explanations. J Biomech 26 Suppl 1:125–136.

Quanbury AO, Winter DA, Reimer GD. 1975. Instantaneous power and power flow in body segments during walking. J Hum Mov Stud 1:59–67.

Renstrom PS, Arms SW, Stanwych TS, Johnson RJ, Pope MH. 1986. Strain within the anterior cruciate ligament during hamstring and quadricep activity. Am J Sports Med 14(1):83–87.

Rivera JE. 1994. Open versus closed kinetic chain rehabilitation of the lower extremity: a functional and biomechanical analysis. J Sport Rehabil 3:154–167.

Robertson DG, Fleming D. 1987. Kinetics of standing broad and vertical jumping. Can J Sport Sci 12:19–23.

Robertson DG, Winter DA. 1980. Mechanical energy generation, absorption and transfer amongst segments during walking. J Biomech 13:845–854.

Roetert EP, Ellenbecker TS. 1998. Complete conditioning for tennis. Champaign, IL: Human Kinetics.

Roetert EP, Garrett GE, Brown SW, Camaione DN. 1992. Performance profiles of nationally ranked junior tennis players. J Appl Sports Sci Res 6:225–231.

Rogol IM, Ernst G, Perrin DH. 1998. Open and closed kinetic chain exercises improve shoulder joint reposition sense equally in healthy subjects. J Athl Training 33(4):315–318.

Rowinski MJ. 1985. Afferent neurobiology of the joint. In: Davies GJ, Gould JA, editors. Orthopaedic and sports physical therapy. St. Louis: Mosby. p. 50–64.

Sachs RA, Daniel DM, Stone ML, Garfein RF. 1989. Patellofemoral problems after anterior cruciate ligament reconstruction. Am J Sports Med 17:760–765.

Saha AK. 1983. Mechanism of shoulder movements and a plea for the recognition of "zero position" of glenohumeral joint [reprinted]. Clin Orthop 173:3–10.

Schaffer SW, Payne ED, Gabbard LR, Garber MB, Halle JS. 1994. Relationship between isokinetic and functional tests of the quadriceps [abstract]. J Orthop Sports Phys Ther 19(1):55.

Schulthies SS, Ricard MD, Alexander KJ, Myrer W. 1998. An electromyographic investigation of 4 elastic tubing closed kinetic chain exercises after anterior cruciate ligament reconstruction. J Athl Training 33(4):328–335.

Silfverskiold JP, Steadman JR, Higgins RW, Hagerman T, Atkins JA. 1988. Rehabilitation of the anterior cruciate ligament in the athlete. Sports Med 6(5):308–319.

Snyder-Mackler L. 1996. Scientific rationale and physiological basis for the use of closed kinetic chain exercise in the lower extremity. J Sport Rehabil 5:2–12.

Snyder-Mackler L, Delitto A, Bailey SL, Stralka SW. 1995. Strength of the quadriceps femoris muscle and functional recovery after reconstruction of the anterior cruciate ligament. J Bone Joint Surg Am 77(8):1166–1173.

Somes S, Worrell TW, Corey B, Ingersol CD. 1997. Effects of patellar taping on patellar position in the open and closed kinetic chain: a preliminary study. J Sport Rehabil 6:299–308.

Steindler A. 1955. Kinesiology of the human body. Springfield, IL: Charles C Thomas.

Steindler A. 1973. Kinesiology of the human body under normal and pathological conditions. Springfield, IL: Charles C Thomas.

Stiene HA, Brosky T, Reinking MF, Nyland J, Mason MB. 1996. A comparison of closed kinetic chain and isokinetic joint isolation exercise in patients with patellofemoral dysfunction. J Orthop Sports Phys Ther 24(3):136–141.

Strizak AM, Gleim GW, Sapega A, Nicholas JA. 1983. Hand and forearm strength and its relation to tennis. Am J Sports Med 11(4):234–239.

Sullivan PE, Markos PD, Minor MAD. 1982. An integrated approach to therapeutic exercise: theory and application. Reston, VA: Reston.

Swarup M, Irrgang JJ, Lephart S. 1992. Relationship of isokinetic quadriceps peak torque and work to one legged hop vertical jump. Phys Ther 72:S88.

Tabor M, Peterson AM, Davies GJ. 1999. Test-retest reliability of the lower extremity functional test [abstract]. Phys Ther 79:S81.

Tegner Y, Lysholm M, Gilquist J. 1986. A performance test to monitor rehabilitation and evaluate anterior cruciate ligament injuries. Am J Sports Med 14:156–159.

Townsend H, Jobe FW, Pink M, Perry J. 1991. Electromyographic analysis of the glenohumeral muscles during a baseball rehabilitation program. Am J Sports Med 19(3):264–272.

VanGheluwe B, Hebbelinck M. 1985. The kinematics of the service movement in tennis: a three dimensional cinematographic approach. In: Winter DA, Norman RW, Biomechanics IX-B. Champaign, IL: Human Kinetics. p. 521–526.

Voight ML, Cook G. 1996. Clinical application of closed kinetic chain exercise. J Sport Rehabil 5(1):25–44.

Warner JJP, Bowen MK, Deng X, Torzilli PA, Warren RF. 1999. Effect of joint compression on inferior stability of the glenohumeral joint. J Shoulder Elbow Surg 8:31–36.

Wawrzyniak JR, Tracy JE, Catizone PV, Storrow RR. 1996. Effect of closed chain exercise on quadriceps femoris peak torque and functional performance. J Athl Training 31(4):335–340.

Weiser WM, Lee TQ, McMaster WC, McMahon PJ. 1999. Effects of simulated scapular protraction on anterior glenohumeral stability. Am J Sports Med 27(6):801–805.

Werner FW, An KN. 1994. Biomechanics of the elbow and forearm. Hand Clin 10:357–373.

Wiklander J, Lysholm J. 1987. Simple tests for surveying muscle strength and muscle stiffness in sportsmen. Int J Sports Med 8:50–54.

Wilk KE, Andrews JR. 1993. The effects of pad placement and angular velocity on tibial displacement during isokinetic exercise. J Orthop Sports Phys Ther 17(1):23–30.

Wilk KE, Andrews JR, Arrigo CA, Keirns MA, Erber DJ. 1993. The strength characteristics of internal and external rotator muscles in professional baseball pitchers. Am J Sports Med 21:61–66.

Wilk KE, Arrigo CA, Andrews JR. 1996. Closed and open kinetic chain exercises for the upper extremity. J Sport Rehabil 5(1):88–102.

Wilk KE, Davies GJ, Mangine RE, Malone TR. 1998. Patellofemoral disorders: a classification system and clinical guidelines for nonoperative rehabilitation. J Orthop Sports Phys Ther 28(5):307–322.

Wilk KE, Escamilla RF, Fleisig GS, Arrigo CA, Barrentine SW. 1995. Open and closed kinetic chain exercise for the lower extremity: theory and clinical application. Athl Training: Sports Health Care Perspect 1(4):336–346.

Wilk KE, Escamilla RF, Flesig GS, Barrentine SW, Andrews JR, Boyd ML. 1996. A comparison of tibiofemoral joint forces and electromyographic activity during open and closed kinetic chain exercises. Am J Sports Med 24(4):518–527.

Wilk KE, Romaniello WT, Soscia SM, Arrigo CA, Andrews JR. 1994. The relationship between subjective knee scores, isokinetic testing and functional testing in the ACL-reconstructed knee. J Orthop Sports Phys Ther 20(2):60–73.

Worrell TW, Borchert B, Erner K, Fritz J, Leerar P. 1993. Effect of a lateral step-up exercise protocol on quadriceps and lower extremity performance. J Orthop Sports Phys Ther 18(6):646–653.

Yack HJ, Collins CE, Whieldon TJ. 1993. Comparisons of closed and open kinetic chain exercise in the anterior cruciate ligament–deficient knee. Am J Sports Med 21(1):49–54.

Zeier FG. 1973. The treatment of winged scapula. Clin Orthop 91:128–133.

Index

Note: The italicized *f* and *t* following a page number indicate figures and tables, respectively.

About the Authors

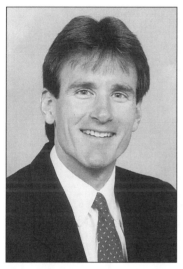

Todd S. Ellenbecker, MS, PT, SCS, OCS, CSCS, is the director of Physiotherapy Associates Scottsdale Sports Clinic, in Scottsdale, Arizona, and is a licensed physical therapist who has researched and taught in the field for 15 years.

The author of *The Elbow in Sport, Complete Conditioning for Tennis,* and *Knee Ligament Rehabilitation,* he has published numerous articles and research studies pertaining to the upper extremity in baseball and tennis players and has treated shoulder and elbow injuries in many professional players.

He is certified by the American Physical Therapy Association (APTA) as both a sports clinical specialist and orthopedic clinical specialist. The APTA also awarded him its Sports Physical Therapy Clinical Teaching Award in 1999. He is chairman of the APTA's Shoulder Special Interest Group and a manuscript reviewer for the *Journal of Orthopaedic and Sports Physical Therapy.*

Ellenbecker earned a bachelor's degree in physical therapy from the University of Wisconsin–La Crosse and a master's degree in exercise physiology from Arizona State University. He also is certified as a strength and conditioning specialist.

Ellenbecker runs and plays tennis in his spare time.

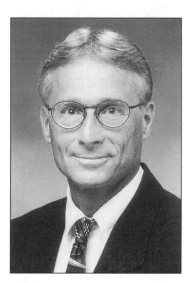

George J. Davies, MEd, PT, SCS, ATC, CSCS, CET, SMAC, has been a professor of physical therapy at the University of Wisconsin–La Crosse graduate physical therapy program for 26 years and presently is the director of clinical and research services at Gundersen Lutheran Sports Medicine-La Crosse, Wisconsin.

Davies has practiced closed kinetic chain exercise for more than 30 years in rehabilitation, performance enhancement, and prevention and has been involved in numerous research studies. He is the author of *A Compendium of Isokinetics in Clinical Usage,* the first book dedicated to the use of isokinetics in clinical settings. He has also published many book chapters and articles in the professional literature.

Davies earned his MEd in health and physical education from Trenton State College and a certificate in physical therapy from the College of Physicians and Surgeons of Columbia University at New York. He also is an ABPTS sports clinical specialist, is certified as an athletic trainer by the NATA, a strength and conditioning specialist by the NSCA, an exercise specialist by the ACSM, and a specialist in martial arts conditioning by the ISSA.

In his leisure time, the former U.S. Marine participates in marathons, triathlons, and weight training and holds a black belt in karate. He has been a sensei (teacher) of karate for several years.

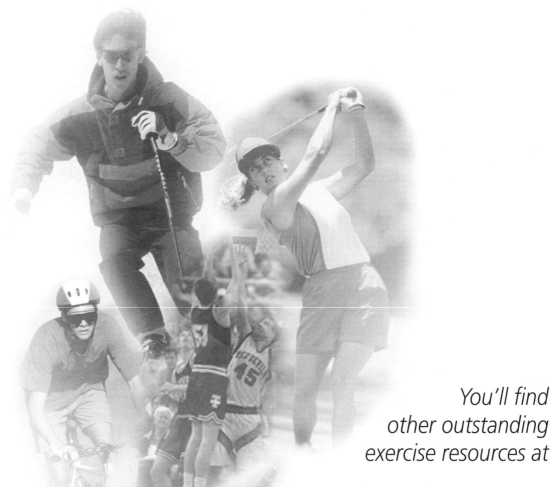